KEY
CHARACTERISTICS
With
COMPARISONS
OF SOME OF THE
LEADING REMEDIES
OF THE
MATERIA MEDICA
WITH BOWEL NOSODES

H.C. ALLEN, M.D.

Eighth Edition

B. Jain Publishers (P) Ltd.
An ISO 9001 : 2000 Certified Company
USA — EUROPE — INDIA

KEYNOTES AND CHARACTERISTICS WITH COMPARISONS

45th Impression: 2010

All rights reserved. No part of this book may be reproduced, stored in a retrieval system or transmitted, in any form or by any means, mechanical, photocopying, recording or otherwise, without any prior written permission of the publisher.

© with the publisher

Published by Kuldeep Jain for

B. JAIN PUBLISHERS (P) LTD.
An ISO 9001 : 2000 Certified Company
1921/10, Chuna Mandi, Paharganj, New Delhi 110 055 (INDIA)
Tel.: 91-11-2358 0800, 2358 1100, 2358 1300, 2358 3100
Fax: 91-11-2358 0471 • *Email:* info@bjain.com
Website: **www.bjainbooks.com**

Printed in India by
J.J. Offset Printers

ISBN: 978-81-319-0349-0

PREFACE: SIXTH EDITION

What applied to former editions applies to this. The fact that a sixth is demanded is convincing proof that Dr. Allen left an indestructible monument of homoeopathic materia medica, one that is true to homoeopathy and immensely helpful to every physician who consults it.

The Publishers

PREFACE: THIRD EDITION

The first edition of this book was only about half the size of the second, as it was prepared somewhat hastily for a special purpose, but Dr. Allen took his time in the second edition, and gave the world a well rounded out and complete standard book on the homoeopathic materia medica. We do not mean that the first edition was faulty as to its matter, for it was used unchanged in the later edition, but it did not embrace a sufficient number of remedies. As Dr. Allen died before a third edition was needed we concluded to bring it out unchanged. It is a masterpiece of materia medica work; its symptomatology is made up of the unchanging landmarks of our remedies that are in constant use; it is, in short, a book that needs no revision.

Philadelphia, Pa.   **The Publishers**

PREFACE: SECOND EDITION

In preparing the second edition for the press the work has been enlarged and practically rewritten. Many more remedies have been included and symptoms and comparisons extended, yet care has been taken that every symptom has been verified. The original plan has been maintained, viz., to give only those symptom—guides that mark the individuality of the remedy, that the student of materia medica may use them as landmarks to master the genius of the remedial agent.

At the suggestion of the publishers and in response to numerous enquiries a more extended symptomatology of the nosodes has been included, for these invaluable additions to our armamentarium, like the so-called tissue remedies of Schüessler, only need more extensive provings to place them in the list of polychrests.

That the student may acquire the correct pronunciation of our remedial agents, an alphabetical list of remedies with the accentuation is given, for a homoeopathic physician may properly be held accountable for the correct use of terms peculiar to his profession. An index of remedies and comparisons is also included.

H.C. Allen

PREFACE: FIRST EDITION

The life work of the student of the homoeopathic materia medica is one of constant comparison and differentiation. He must compare the pathogenesis of a remedy with the recorded anamnesis of the patient; he must differentiate the apparently similar symptoms of two or more medicinal agents in order to select the similimum. To enable the student or practitioner to do this correctly and rapidly he must have as a basis for comparison some knowledge of the individuality of the remedy; something that is peculiar, uncommon, or sufficiently characteristic in the confirmed pathogenesis of a polychrest remedy that may be a so-called "keynote," a "characteristic," the "red strand of the rope," and central modality or principle—as the aggravation from motion of Bryonia, the amelioration from motion of Rhus, the furious, vicious delirium of Belladonna or the apathetic indifference of Phosphoric acid—some familiar landmark around which the symptoms may be arranged in the mind for comparison.

Something of this kind seems indispensable to enable us to intelligently and successfully use our voluminous symptomatology. Also, if we may judge from the small number of homoeopathic physicians who rely on the single remedy in practice, and the almost constant demand for a "revision" of the materia medica, its study in the past, as well as at present, has not been altogether satisfactory to the majority.

An attempt to render the student's task less difficult, to simplify its study, to make it both interesting and useful, to place its mastery within the reach of every intelligent man or woman in the profession, is the apology for the addition of another monograph to our present works of reference.

It is all important that the first step in the study of homoeopathic therapeutics be correctly taken, for the pathway is then more direct and the view more comprehensive. The object of this work is to and the student to master that which is guiding and characteristic in the individuality of each remedy and thus utilize more readily the symptomatology of the homoeopathic materia medica, the most comprehensive and practical work for the cure of the sick ever given the medical practitioner and teacher, and is published at the earnest solicitation of many alumni of Hering College, with the hope that it may be of as much benefit to the beginner as it has been to the compiler.

H. C. Allen

CONTENTS

ALPHABETICAL LIST OF REMEDIES

Abrotanum	1
Aceticum acidum	2
Aconitum napellus	3
Actaea racemosa	6
Aesculus hippocastanum	8
Aethusa cynapium	10
Agaricus muscarius	11
Agnus castus	13
Allium cepa	14
Aloe Socotrina	16
Alumina	18
Ambra grisea	20
Ammonium carbonicum	21
Ammonium muriaticum	23
Amylenum nitrosum	24
Anacardium orientale	26
Anthracinum	28
Antimonium crudum	29
Antimonium tartaricum	32
Apis mellifica	34
Apocynum cannabinum	36
Argentum metallicum	37
Argentum nitricum	39
Arnica montana	41
Arsenicum album	44
Arum triphyllum	47
Asarum europaeum	49

Asterias rubens 50
Aurum metallicum 51
Baptisia tinctoria 54
Baryta carbonica 55
Belladonna 57
Benzoicum acidum 60
Berberis vulgaris 61
Bismuthum 62
Borax 63
Bovista 65
Bromium 66
Bryonia alba 68
Cactus grandiflorus 71
Caladium 72
Calcarea arsenicosa 73
Calcarea ostrearum 73
Calcarea phosphorica 76
Calendula 78
Camphora officinalis 80
Cannabis indica 81
Cannabis sativa 82
Cantharides 83
Capsicum 85
Carbo animalis 86
Carbo vegetabilis 88
Carbolicum acidum 90
Caulophyllum 92
Causticum 93
Chamomilla 96
Chelidonium majus 98
Cicuta virosa 100

Cina maritima	101
Cinchona	103
Coca	105
Cocculus	106
Coffea cruda	108
Colchicum autumnale	109
Collinsonia canadensis	111
Colocynthis	112
Conium maculatum	113
Crocus sativus	116
Crotalus horridus	117
Croton tiglium	119
Cuprum metallicum	120
Cyclamen europaeum	122
Digitalis purpurea	124
Dioscorea villosa	125
Diphtherinum	126
Drosera rotundifolia	128
Dulcamara	130
Equisetum hyemale	132
Eupatorium perfoliatum	132
Euphrasia	134
Ferrum metallicum	135
Fluoricum acidum	137
Gelsemium	138
Glonoinum	140
Graphites	142
Hamamelis virginica	144
Helleborus niger	146
Helonias dioica	148
Hepar sulphuris	149

Hydrastis canadensis 152
Hyoscyamus niger 152
Hypericum perforatum 154
Ignatia 156
Iodium 158
Ipecacuanha 160
Kalium bichromicum 162
Kalium bromatum 165
Kalium carbonicum 166
Kalmia latifolia 168
Kreosotum 169
Lachesis 171
Lac caninum 175
Lac defloratum 178
Ledum palustre 179
Lilium tigrinum 181
Lobelia inflata 183
Lycopodium clavatum 185
Lyssinum 188
Magnesium carbonicum 189
Magnesium muriaticum 191
Magnesium phosphoricum 193
Medorrhinum 195
Melilotus alba 201
Menyanthes trifoliata 202
Mercurius 203
Mercurius biniodatus 206
Mercurius corrosivus 207
Mercurius cyanatus 207
Mercurius dulcis 208
Mercurius proto-iodatus 208

Mercurius solubilis	209
Mercurius sulphuricus	210
Mezereum	211
Millefolium	212
Murex purpurea	213
Muriaticum acidum	214
Naja tripudians	216
Natrium carbonicum	217
Natrium muriaticum	218
Natrium sulphuricum	222
Nitricum acidum	224
Nux moschata	227
Nux vomica	230
Opium	233
Petroleum	236
Petroselinum	238
Phosphoricum acidum	239
Phosphorus	241
Physostigma	244
Phytolacca decandra	245
Picricum acidum	247
Platinum	248
Plumbum	250
Podophyllum	252
Psorinum	254
Pulsatilla	258
Pyrogenium	261
Ratanhia	263
Ranunculus bulbosus	264
Rheum	265
Rhododendron	266

- Rhus toxicodendron 267
- Rumex crispus 270
- Ruta graveolens 272
- Sabadilla 273
- Sabina 274
- Sambucus nigra 276
- Sanguinaria 277
- Sanicula 279
- Sarsaparilla 281
- Secale cornutum 283
- Selenium 285
- Sepia 287
- Silicea 291
- Spigelia 295
- Spongia tosta 297
- Stannum 298
- Staphysagria 300
- Stramonium 303
- Sulphur 306
- Sulphuricum acidum 310
- Symphytum 312
- Syphilinum 312
- Tabacum 315
- Taraxacum 317
- Tarentula 318
- Terebinthiniae 320
- Theridion curassavicum 321
- Thlaspi bursa pastoris 323
- Thuja occidentalis 323
- Trillium pendulum 327
- Tuberculinum – bacillinum* 328

Valeriana 330
Variolinum 331
Veratrum album 332
Veratrum viride 335
Zincum metallicum 336

MATERIA MEDICA OF SOME MORE IMPORTANT REMEDIES

Adrenalinum (sarcode) 341
Bacillinum 345
Cholesterinum 348
Electricitas 350
Electricity 351
Lac felinum 358
Lac vaccinum 363
Magnetis poli ambo 366
Magnetis polus arcticus 376
Magnetis polus australis 386
Malandrinum 394
Malaria officinalis 401
Thyroidinum 409
Ustilago 416
Vaccininum 430
Provings of the X-ray 434
The bowel nosodes 445
   Introduction 445
   Morgan (Bach) 450
   Proteus (Bach) 453
   Bacillus No. "7" (Paterson) 456
   Gaertner (Bach) 457

Dys. Co. (Bach) 458
Sycotic Co. (Paterson) 460
Mutabile (Bach) 463
Faecalis (Bach) 463
B. Morgan (Bach) 464
B. Proteus (Bach) 464
Bacillus No. "7" (Paterson) 464
B. Gaertner (Bach) 464
The bowel nosodes 470
Index 473

ABROTANUM

Southernwood   *Compositae*

Alternate constipation and diarrhea; lienteria.

Marasmus of children with marked emaciation, especially of legs (Iod., Sanic., Tub.); the skin is flabby and hangs loose in folds (of neck, Nat-m., Sanic.).

In marasmus, head weak, cannot hold it up (Aeth.).

Marasmus of lower extremities only.

Ravenous hunger; losing flesh while eating well (Iod., Nat-m., Sanic., Tub.).

Painful contractions of the limbs from cramps or following colic.

Rheumatism; for the excessive pain before the swelling commences; from suddenly checked diarrhea or other secretions; alternates with hemorrhoids, with dysentery.

Gout; joints stiff, swollen, with pricking sensation; wrists and ankle joints painful and inflamed.

Very lame and sore all over.

Itching chilblains (Agar.).

Great weakness and prostration and a kind of hectic fever with children; unable to stand.

Child is ill-natured, irritable, cross and despondent; violent, inhuman, would like to do something cruel.

Face old, pale, wrinkled (Op.).

Relationship

After Hepar in furuncle; after Acon. and Bry. in pleurisy, when a pressing sensation remains in affected side impeding respiration.

ACETICUM ACIDUM

Glacial Acetic Acid $C_4H_3O_3$

Adapted to pale, lean persons with lax, flabby muscles; *face pale, waxy* (Ferr.).

Hemorrhage: From every mucous outlet, nose, throat, lungs, stomach, bowels, uterus (Ferr., Mill.); metrorrhagia; vicarious; traumatic epistaxis (Arn.).

Marasmus and other wasting diseases of children (Abrot., Iod., Sanic., Tub.).

Great prostration; after injuries (Sul-ac.); *after surgical shock; after anesthetics.*

Thirst: Intense, burning, insatiable even for large quantities in dropsy, diabetes, chronic diarrhea; **but no thirst in fever.**

Sour belching and vomiting of pregnancy, burning waterbrash and profuse salivation, day and night (Lac-ac.; salivation, < at night, Merc.).

Diarrhea: Copious, exhausting, great thirst; in dropsy, typhus, phthisis; with night sweats.

True croup, hissing respiration, cough with the inhalation (Spong.); last stages.

Inhalation of vapor of cider vinegar has been successfully used in croup and malignant diphtheria.

Cannot sleep lying on the back (sleeps better on back, Ars.); sensation of sinking in abdomen causing dyspnea; *rests better lying on belly* (Am-c.).

Hectic fever, skin dry and hot; *red spot on left cheek and drenching night sweats.*

Relationship

It antidotes anesthetic vapors (Aml-ns.); fumes of charcoal and gas; Opium and Stramonium.

Cider vinegar antidotes Carbolic acid.

Follows well: After Cinchona, in hemorrhage; after Digitalis in dropsy.

It aggravates: The symptoms of Arn., Bell., Lach., Merc.; especially the headache from Belladonna.

ACONITUM NAPELLUS

Monkshood *Ranunculaceae*

Is generally indicated in acute or recent cases occurring in young persons, especially girls of a full, plethoric habit *who lead a sedentary life;* persons easily affected by atmospheric changes; dark hair and eyes, rigid muscular fibre.

Complaints caused by exposure to *dry cold air, dry north* or *west winds,* or exposure to draughts of cold air while in a perspiration; bad effects of checked perspiration.

Great fear and anxiety of mind, with great nervous excitability; afraid to go out, to go into a crowd where there is any excitement or many people; to cross the street.

The countenance is expressive of **fear;** *the life is rendered miserable by fear;* is sure his disease will prove fatal; predicts the day he will die; fear of death during pregnancy.

Restless, anxious, does everything in great haste; must change position often; everything startles him.

Pains: Are intolerable, they drive him crazy; he becomes very restless; at night.

Hahnemann says: "Whenever Aconite is chosen homoeopathically, you must, above all, observe the moral symptoms, and be careful that it closely resembles them; the anguish of mind and body; the restlessness; the disquiet not to be allayed."

This mental anxiety, worry, fear accompanies the most trivial ailment.

Music is unbearable, makes her sad (Sab.; during menses, Nat-c.).

On rising from a recumbent position the red face becomes deathly pale, or he becomes faint or giddy and

ACONITUM NAPELLUS

falls, and he fears to rise again; often accompanied by vanishing of sight and unconsciousness.

Amenorrhea in plethoric young girls; **after fright,** to prevent suppression of menses.

For the congestive stage of inflammation before localization takes place.

Fever: **Skin dry and hot;** face red, or pale and red alternately; *burning thirst for large quantities of cold water;* **intense nervous restlessness, tossing about in agony;** becomes intolerable towards evening and on going to sleep.

Convulsions: Of teething children; heat, jerks and twitches of single muscles; child gnaws its fist, frets and screams; skin hot and dry; high fever.

Cough, croup; dry, hoarse, suffocating; loud, rough, croaking; hard, ringing, whistling; on *expiration* (Caust.; on inhalation, Spong.); **from dry, cold winds or drafts of air.**

Aconite should never be given simply to control the fever, never alternated with other drugs for that purpose. If it be a case requiring Aconite no other drug is needed; Aconite will cure the case.

Unless indicated by the exciting cause, is nearly always injurious in first stages of typhoid fever.

Relationship

Complementary: To Coffea in fever, sleeplessness, intolerance of pain; to Arnica in traumatism; to Sulphur in all cases. Rarely indicated in fevers which bring out eruptions.

Aconite is the acute of Sulphur, and both precede and follow it in acute inflammatory conditions.

Aggravation

Evening and night, pains are insupportable; in a warm room; when rising from bed; lying on affected side (Hep., Nux-m.).

Amelioration

In the open air (Alum., Mag-c., Puls., Sab.).

ACTAEA RACEMOSA

Black Cohosh　　　　　　　　　　***Ranunculaceae***

Puerperal mania; thinks she is going crazy (compare, Syph.); tries to injure herself.

Mania following disappearance of neuralgia.

Sensation as if a *heavy, black cloud settled all over her and enveloped her* head so that all is darkness and confusion.

Illusion of a mouse running from under her chair (Lac-c., Aeth.).

Ciliary neuralgia: Aching or sharp, darting, shooting pains in globes, extending to temples, vertex, occiput, orbit, < going up stairs, > lying down.

Heart troubles from reflex symptoms of uterus or ovaries. Heart's action ceases suddenly; impending suffocation; palpitation from least motion (Dig.).

ACTAEA RACEMOSA

Menses: Irregular; exhausting (Alum., Cocc.); delayed or suppressed by mental emotion, from cold, from fever; with chorea, hysteria or mania; increase of mental symptoms during.

Spasms: Hysterical or epileptic; reflex from uterine disease; worse during menses; chorea < left side.

Severe left-sided inframammary pains (Ust.).

Sharp, lancinating electric-like pains in various parts, sympathetic with ovarian or uterine irritation; in uterine region, dart from side to side.

Pregnancy; *nausea;* sleeplessness; *false labor-like pains;* sharp pains across abdomen; abortion at third month (Sab.).

During labor: *"shivers" in first stage;* convulsions, from nervous excitement; rigid os; pains severe, spasmodic, tedious, < by least noise.

After-pains, worse in the groins.

When given during last month of pregnancy shortens labor, if symptoms correspond (Caul., Puls.).

Excessive muscular soreness, after dancing, skating, or other violent muscular exertion.

Rheumatic pains in muscles of neck and back; feel stiff, lame, contracted; spine sensitive, from using arms in sewing, typewriting, piano playing (Agar., Ran-b.).

Rheumatism affecting the bellies of the muscles; pains, stitching, cramping.

Rheumatic dysmenorrhea.

Relationship

Similar: To, Caul. and Puls. in uterine and rheumatic affections; to, Agar., Lil-t., Sep.

Aggravation

During menstruation: The more profuse the flow the greater the suffering.

AESCULUS HIPPOCASTANUM

Horse Chestnut   *Sapindaceae*

For persons with hemorrhoidal tendencies, and who suffer with gastric, bilious or catarrhal troubles.

Fullness in various parts, as from an undue amount of blood; heart, lungs, stomach, brain, pelvis, skin.

Venous congestion, especially portal and hemorrhoidal.

Despondent, gloomy; very irritable; loses temper easily and gains control slowly; *miserably cross* (Cham.).

Mucous membranes of mouth, throat, rectum are swollen, burn, feel dry and raw.

Coryza: Thin, watery, burning; rawness and sensitive to inhaled cold air.

Follicular pharyngitis: Violent burning, raw sensation in throat; dryness and roughness of throat.

Frequent inclination to swallow, with burning, pricking, stinging and dry constricted fauces (Apis, Bell.).

AESCULUS HIPPOCASTANUM

Rectum: *Dryness and heat of;* feels as if *full of small sticks;* knife-like pains shoot up the rectum (Ign., Sulph.); hemorrhoids blind, painful, burning, purplish, rarely bleeding.

Rectum sore, with fullness, burning and itching (Sulph.).

Constipation: Hard, dry stool, difficult to pass; with dryness and heat of rectum; *severe lumbo-sacral backache.*

Stool followed by *fullness of rectum and intense pain in anus* for hours (Aloe, Ign., Mur-ac., Sulph.).

Prolapsus uteri and acrid, dark leucorrhea, with lumbo-sacral backache and great fatigue, from walking.

Severe dull backache in lumbo-sacral articulation; more or less constant; affecting sacrum and hips.

Back "gives out": During pregnancy, prolapsus, leucorrhea; when walking or stooping; must sit or lie down.

Sensation of heaviness and lameness in back.

Paralytic feeling in arms, legs and spine.

Relationship

Similar: To, Aloe, Coll., Ign., Mur-ac., Nux-v., Sulph., in hemorrhoids.

After Coll. has improved piles, Aesc. often cures.

Useful after Nux-v. and Sulph. have improved, but failed to cure piles.

Aggravation

Motion; backache and soreness by walking and stooping; inhaling cold air.

AETHUSA CYNAPIUM

Fool's Parsley   *Umbelliferae*

Especially for children during dentition in hot summer weather; **children who cannot bear milk.**

Great weakness: Children cannot stand; unable to hold up the head (Abrot.); prostration with sleepiness.

Idiocy in children; incapacity to think; confused.

An expression of great anxiety and pain, with a drawn condition and well-marked linea nasalis.

Features expressive of pain and anxiety.

Herpetic eruption on end of the nose.

Complete absence of thirst (Apis, Puls.—rev. of Ars.).

Intolerance of milk: *Cannot bear milk in any form;* it is vomited in large curds as soon as taken; then weakness causes drowsiness (compare, Mag-c.).

Indigestion of teething children; *violent, sudden vomiting* of a frothy; milk-white substance; or yellow fluid, *followed by curdled milk and cheesy matter.*

Regurgitation of food an hour or so after eating; copious greenish vomiting.

Epileptic spasms, with *clenched thumbs*, red face, **eyes turned downwards,** pupils fixed and dilated; foam at the mouth, jaws locked; pulse small, hard, quick.

Weakness and prostration with sleepiness; after vomiting, after stool, after spasm.

Relationship

Similar: To, Ant-c., Ars., Calc., Sanic.

Aggavation

After eating or drinking; after vomiting; after stool; after spasm.

AGARICUS MUSCARIUS

Toadstool *Fungi*

Person with light hair; skin and muscles lax.

Old people, with weak, indolent circulation.

Drunkards, especially for their headaches; *bad effects after a debauch* (Lob., Nux-v., Ran-b.).

Delirium: With constant raving; tries to get out of bed; in typhoid or typhus.

Headaches: Of those who readily become delirious in fever or with pain (Bell.); of persons subject to chorea, twitchings or grimaces; from spinal affections.

Chilblains, that itch and burn intolerably; frostbite and all consequences of exposure to cold, especially in face.

Involuntary movements *while awake,* cease during sleep; chorea, from simple motions and jerks of single muscles to dancing of whole body; trembling of whole body (twitching of muscles of face, Mygal.).

Sensation as if ice touched or ice-cold needles were piercing the skin; as from hot needles.

Burning, itching, redness of various parts; ears, nose, face, hands and feet; parts red, swollen, hot.

Uncertainty in walking, stumbling gait, stumbles over everything in the way; feels pain as if beaten, when standing.

Spine sensitive to touch (Ther.); worse mornings.

Pain: Sore, aching, in lumbar and sacral regions; during exertion in the day time; *while sitting* (Zinc.).

Spinal irritation due to sexual excesses (Kali-p.).

Nervous prostration after sexual debauches.

Epilepsy from suppressed eruptions (Psor., Sulph.).

Every motion, every turn of body, causes pain in, spine. Single vertebra sensitive to touch.

Prolapsus, post-climacteric; bearing-down pain almost intolerable (compare, Lilium, Murex, Sepia.).

Extremely sensitive to cold air (Calc., Kali-c., Psor.).

Complaints appear diagonally; upper left and lower right side (Ant-t., Stram.—upper right, lower left, Ambr., Brom., Med., Phos., Sul-ac.).

Relationship

Similar: To, Cimic., Calc., Cann-i., Ind., Hyos., Kali-p., Lach., Nux-v., Op., Stram., in delirium of alcoholism; to Mygal., Tarent., Zinc., in chorea.

Aggavation

After eating; after coitus; cold air; mental application; before a thunderstorm (Phos., Psor.).

AGNUS CASTUS

Chaste Tree   *Verbenaceae*

For the lymphatic constitution.

Absent-minded, reduced power of insight; cannot recollect; has to read a sentence twice before he can comprehend (Lyc., Ph-ac., Sep.).

"Old sinners," with impotence and gleet; unmarried persons suffering from nervous debility.

Premature old age: Melancholy, apathy, mental distraction, self-contempt; arising in young persons from abuse of the sexual powers; from seminal losses.

Complete impotence: Relaxation, flaccidity, coldness of genitalia. No sexual power or desire (Calad., Sel.).

Impotence, after frequent attacks of gonorrhea.

Bad effects from suppressed gonorrhea (Med.).

Gleet, with absence of sexual desire or erections.

Leucorrhea; transparent, but staining linen yellow; passes imperceptibly *from the very relaxed parts.*

Deficient secretion or suppression of milk in nursing women (Asaf., Lac-c., Lac-d.); often with great sadness; says she will die.

Complaints of imaginary odor before the nose, as of hering or musk.

Prevents excoriation, from walking.

Relationship

Calad. and Sel. follow well after Agnus in weakness of sexual organs or impotence.

ALLIUM CEPA

Onion   *Liliaceae*

Acute catarrhal inflammation of mucous membranes, with increased secretion.

Catarrhal dull headache, with coryza; < in the evening, > in open air; < on returning to a warm room (compare, Euphr., Puls.).

Headache ceases during menses; returns when flow disappears (Lach., Zinc.).

Eyes: Burning, biting, smarting as from smoke, must rub them; watery and suffused; capillaries injected and excessive lachrymation.

Coryza: *Profuse, watery and acrid nasal discharge*, with profuse, bland lachrymation (profuse, full of acrid tears, bland and fluent coryza, Euphr.).

Acrid, watery discharge dropping from tip of nose (Ars., Ars-i.).

Spring coryza: After damp northeasterly winds; discharge burns and corrodes nose and upper lip.

Hay fever: In August every year; violent sneezing on rising from bed; from handling peaches.

Nasal polypus (Teucr., Sang., Sangin-n., Psor.).

Catarrhal laryngitis; cough compels patient to *grasp the larynx*; seems as *if cough would tear it.*

Colic: From cold by getting feet wet; overeating; from cucumbers; salads; hemorrhoidal; of children; < sitting, > moving about.

Neuralgic pains like a long thread; in face, head, neck, chest.

Traumatic chronic neuritis; neuralgia of stump after amputation; burning and stinging pains.

Panaritia; with red streaks up the arm; pains drive to despair; in child-bed.

Sore and raw spots on feet, especially heel, from *friction.* "*Efficacious when feet are rubbed sore.*" — Dioscorides.

Phlebitis, puerperal; after forceps delivery.

Relationship

Complementary: Phos., Puls., Thuj.

Compatible: Before, Calc. and Sil. in polypus.

Similar: To, Euphr., but coryza and lachrymation are opposite.

Bad effects from getting wet (Rhus-t.).

Aggravation

Predominantly in the evening and in warm room (Puls.; in open air, Euphr.).

Amelioration

In cold room and *open air* (Puls.).

ALOE SOCOTRINA

Socotrine Aloes *Liliaceae*

Adapted to indolent, "weary", persons; averse to either mental or physical labor; mental labor fatigues.

Old people; especially women of relaxed, phlegmatic habit. Extreme prostration, with perspiration.

Itch appears each year, as winter approaches (Psor.).

Dissatisfied and angry about himself or his complaints, especially when constipated.

Diseases of mucous membranes; causes the production of *mucus in jelly-like lumps* from throat or rectum; affects mucous membrane of rectum.

Headache across the forehead < by every footstep (Bell., Bry.); with heaviness of eyes and nausea.

Headaches: Are worse from heat, better from cold applications (Ars.); alternating with lumbago; after insufficient stool.

Diarrhea: Has to hurry to closet *immediately* after *eating and drinking* (Crot-t.); *with want of confidence in sphincter ani; driving out of bed early in the morning* (Psor., Rumx., Sulph.).

When passing flatus, sensation as if stool would pass with it (Olnd., Mur-ac., Nat-m.).

Colic: Cutting, griping pain in right lower portion of abdomen; excruciating, *before and during stool*; all pains cease after stool, leaving profuse sweating and

ALOE SOCOTRINA

extreme weakness; *attacks preceded by obstinate constipation.*

Flatus offensive, burning, copious; much flatus with small stool (Agar.); burning in anus after passage of flatus.

Solid stool and masses of mucus pass involuntarily; hungry during diarrhea.

Before stool: Rumbling, violent sudden urging, *heaviness in rectum;* during stool, tenesmus and *much flatus;* after stool, faintness.

Hemorrhoids: Blue, like a bunch of grapes (Mur-ac.); constant bearing down in rectum; bleeding, sore, tender, hot, relieved by cold water; intense itching.

Itching and burning in anus, preventing sleep (Indg.).

Relationship

Like Sulphur in many chronic diseases with abdominal plethora and congestion of portal circulation; develops suppressed eruptions.

Similar: To, Am-m., Gamb., Nux-v., Podo.

Aggravation

Early morning; sedentary life; *hot, dry weather;* after eating or drinking; standing or walking.

Amelioration

Cold water; cold weather; discharge of flatus and stool.

ALUMINA

Pure Clay Al_2O_3

Adapted to persons who suffer from chronic diseases; "the Aconite of chronic diseases."

Constitutions deficient in animal heat (Calc., Sil.).

Spare, dry, thin subjects; dark complexion; mild, cheerful disposition; hypochondriacs; dry, tettery, itching eruption, worse in winter (Petr.); intolerable, itching of whole body when getting warm in bed (Sulph.); scratches until bleeds, then becomes painful.

Time passes too slowly; an hour seems half a day (Cann-i.)

Inability to walk, except with the eyes open, and in the daytime; tottering and falling when closing eyes (Arg-n., Gels.).

Abnormal appetite; craving for starch, chalk, charcoal, cloves, coffee or tea-grounds, acids and indigestible things (Cic., Psor.); *potatoes disagree.*

Chronic eructations for years; worse in evening.

All irritating things—salt, wine, vinegar, pepper— immediately produce cough.

Constipation: *No desire for and no ability to pass stool until there is a large accumulation* (Meli-a.); **great straining,** must grasp the seat of closet tightly; stool hard, knotty, like laurel berries, covered with mucus; or soft, clayey, adhering to parts (Plat.).

ALUMINA

Inactivity of rectum, *even soft stool requires great straining* (Anac., Puls., Sil., Verat.).

Constipation: Of nursing children, from artificial food; bottle-fed babies; of old people (Lyc., Op.); of pregnancy, from inactive rectum (Sep.).

Diarrhea when she urinates.

Has to strain at stool in order to urinate.

Leucorrhea: **Acrid and profuse, running down to the heels** (Syph.); worse during the daytime; > by cold bathing.

After menses: *Exhausted physically and mentally,* scarcely able to speak (Carb-an., Cocc.).

Talking fatigues; faint and tired, must sit down.

Relationship

Complementary: To, Bryonia.

Follows: Bry., Lach., Sulph.

Alumina is the chronic of Bryonia.

Similar: To, Bar-c., Con., in ailments of old people.

Aggravation

In cold air; during winter; while sitting; *from eating potatoes;* after eating soups; on alternate days; *at new and full moon.*

Amelioration

Mild summer weather; from warm drinks; *while eating* (Psor.); in wet weather (Caust.).

Alumina is one of the chief antidotes for lead poisoning; painter's colic; ailments from lead.

AMBRA GRISEA

Ambergris   *A Nosode*

For children, especially young girls who are excitable, nervous and weak; nervous affections of old people, nerves "worn out."

Lean, thin, emaciated persons who take cold easily.

Great sadness, sits for days weeping.

After business embarrassments, unable to sleep, must get up (Cimic., Sep.).

Ranula with fetid breath (Thuj.).

Sensation of coldness in abdomen (Calc.).

The presence of others, even the nurse, is unbearable during stool; frequent, ineffectual desire, which makes her anxious.

Discharge of blood between periods, at every little accident a long walk, after every hard stool, etc.

Leucorrhea: *Thick, bluish-white mucus,* especially or only at night (Caust., Merc., Nit-ac.).

Violent cough in spasmodic paroxysms, with eructations and hoarseness; worse talking or reading aloud (Dros., Phos.); evening without, morning with expectoration (Hyos.); whooping cough, but without crowing inspiration.

Relationship

Similar: To, Asaf., Cimic., Coca, Ign., Mosch., Phos., Valer.

Aggravation

Warm drinks, warm room; music; lying down; reading or talking aloud; the presence of many people; after waking.

Amelioration

After eating; cold air; cold food and drinks; rising from bed.

AMMONIUM CARBONICUM

Smelling Salts $\qquad$ $2NH_4O.\ 3CO_2$

Hemorrhagic diathesis, fluid blood and degeneration of red blood corpuscles; ulcerations tend to gangrene.

Stout, fleshy women with various troubles in consequence of leading a sedentary life; delicate women who must have the "smelling bottle" continually at hand; readily catch cold in winter.

Children dislike washing (Ant-c., Sulph.).

Loses breath when falling asleep, must awaken to get breath (Grin., Lach.).

Ill-humor during wet, stormy weather.

Headache; sensation of fullness, as if forehead would burst (Bell., Glon.).

Nosebleed: **When washing the face** (Arn., Mag-c.) and hands in the morning, from left nostril; *after eating*.

AMMONIUM CARBONICUM

Ozena, blowing bloody mucus from the nose frequently; blood rushes to tip of nose, when stooping.

Stopping of nose, mostly at night; *must breathe through the mouth,* a keynote even in diphtheria; long lasting coryza; "snuffles" of infants (Hep., Nux-v., Samb., Stict.).

Putrid sore throat; tendency to gangrenous ulceration of tonsils; glands engorged.

In diphtheria or scarlatina when *the nose is stopped up;* child cannot sleep because it cannot get its breath.

Cholera-like symptoms at the commencement of menstruation (Bov., Verat.).

Menses: Too early, profuse, preceded by griping colic; acrid, makes the thighs sore; copious at night and when sitting (Zinc.); with toothache, colic, sadness; *fatigue,* especially of thighs; yawning and chilliness.

Leucorrhea: Watery, burning from the uterus; acrid, profuse from the vagina; excoriation of vulva.

Dyspnea with palpitation, worse by exertion or on ascending even a few steps; worse in a warm room.

One of the best remedies in emphysema.

Cough: Dry, from tickling in throat as from dust, every morning from 3 to 4 a.m. (Kali-c.).

Panaritium: Deep-seated periosteal pain (Dios., Sil.).

Body red, as if from scarlatina (compare, Ail.).

Malignant scarlatina with deep sleep; stertorous breathing. Miliary rash or faintly developed eruption from defective vitality; threatened paralysis of brain (Tub., Zinc.).

Relationship

It antidotes, poisoning with Rhus and stings of insects.

Affects the right side most.

Inimical: To, Lachesis.

Aggravation

Cold, wet weather; wet poultices; from washing; during menses.

Amelioration

Lying on abdomen (Acet-ac.); on painful side (Puls.); in dry weather.

AMMONIUM MURIATICUM

Sal Ammoniac NH_4Cl

Especially adapted to those who are fat and sluggish; or *body large and fat, but legs too thin.*

Watery, acrid coryza, corroding the lip (All-c.).

During menses: *Diarrhea and vomiting, bloody discharge from the bowels* (Phos.); neuralgic pains in the feet; flow more profuse at night (Bov.; on lying down, Kreos.).

Obstinate constipation accompanied by much flatus.

Hard, crumbling stools require great effort in expulsion; crumble from the verge of anus (Mag-m.);

vary in color, no two stools alike (Puls.).

Hemorrhoids: Sore and smarting; with burning and stinging in the rectum for hours after stool (Aesc., Sulph.); especially after suppressed leucorrhea.

Leucorrhea: Like white of egg, preceded by griping pain about the navel; brown, slimy, painless, *after every urination*.

Sensation of coldness in the back, between scapulae (Lachn.).

Hamstrings feel painfully short when walking; tension in joints as from shortening of the muscles (Caust., Cimx.).

Offensive sweat of the feet (Alum., Graph., Psor., Sanic., Sil.).

Relationship

Followed: By, Ant-c., Phos., Puls., Sanic.

AMYLENUM NITROSUM

Nitrite of Amyl $C_{10}H_{11}O_2NO_3$

For nervous, sensitive, plethoric women, during or after the menopause.

Often palliative in incurable cases; very important as regards euthanasia.

Rapidly dilates the arteries and accelerates, but later weakens and retards the pulse.

Intense surging of blood to face and head (Bell., Glon.).

Craves fresh air; opens clothing, removes bed covering and opens windows in the coldest weather (Arg-n., Lach., Sulph.).

Flushings: Start from face, stomach, various parts of body, followed by sweating, often hot, profuse; abruptly limited, parts below are icy cold; followed by great prostration.

Face flushes at the slightest emotion (Coca, Ferr.).

Blushing: Chronic or acute. *Sea sickness.*

Hemicrania, especially when afflicted side is pallid.

Collar seems too tight, must loosen it (Lach.).

Angina pectoris: Tumultuous heart action; intense throbbing of heart and carotids (Glon.).

Constant stretching for hours; impossible to satisfy the desire; would seize the bed and call for help to stretch.

Profound and repeated yawning (Kali-c.).

Puerperal convulsions immediately after delivery.

Relationship

Similar: To, Bell., Cact., Coca, Ferr., Glon., Lach.

Aggravation

Mental or physical exertion.

Acts promptly by inhalation; resuscitates persons sinking under anesthetics.

Crude drug chiefly palliative; must be repeated as

patient becomes accustomed to it; *is curative* in the stronger higher potencies.

The cure more frequently depends upon the strength of the potency than many who have not put it to the curative test imagine.

ANACARDIUM ORIENTALE

Marking Nut *Anacardiaceae*

Sudden loss of memory; everything seems to be in a dream; patient is greatly troubled about his forgetfulness; confused, unfit for business.

Disposed to be malicious, seems bent on wickedness.

Irresistible desire to curse and swear (Lac-c., Lil-t., Nit-ac.; wants to *pray* continually, Stram.).

Lack of confidence in himself and others.

Feels as though he had two wills, one commanding him to do what the other forbids.

When walking, is anxious, as if someone were pursuing him; suspects everything around him.

Weakness of all the senses.

Hypochondriac, with hemorrhoids and constipation.

Strange temper, laughs at serious matters and is serious over laughable things. Thinks herself a demon; curses and swears.

Sensation: As of a hoop or band around a part (Cact., Carb-ac., Sulph.); or as of a dull, blunt instrument pressing; as of a plug in inner parts.

Headache: *Relieved entirely when eating* (Psor.); when lying down in bed at night, and when about falling asleep; worse during motion and work.

Gastric and nervous headaches of sedentary persons (Arg-n., Bry., Nux-v.).

Apt to choke when eating and drinking (Cann-s., Nit-ac., Pip-m.).

Swallows food and drink hastily; symptoms disappear while eating (Kali-p., Psor.).

Stomach: Sensation of fasting "all gone," comes on only when stomach is empty and *is > by eating* (Chel., Iod.); > during process of digestion (rev. of Bry., Nux-v.).

Warts on palms of hands (Nat-m.).

Great desire for stool, but with the effort the desire passes away without evacuation; rectum seems powerless, paralyzed, with sensation as if plugged up (irregular peristaltic or over action, Nux-v.).

Relationship

Compare: Rhus-r., Rhus-t. and Rhus-v.

Symptoms are prone to go from right to left (Lyc.).

Anacardium follows well: After Lyc. and Puls.

Anacardium follows, and is followed by Platina.

ANTHRACINUM

Anthrax Poison   *A Nosode*

In carbuncle, malignant ulcer and complaints with *ulceration, sloughing and intolerable burning*.

When Arsenicum or the best selected remedy fails to relieve the burning pain of carbuncle or malignant ulceration.

Hemorrhages: Blood oozes from mouth, nose, anus or sexual organs; black, thick, tar-like, rapidly decomposing (Crot-t.).

Septic fever, rapid loss of strength, sinking pulse, delirium and fainting (Pyrog.).

Gangrenous ulcers; felon, carbuncle, erysipelas of a malignant type.

Felon; the worst cases, with sloughing and terrible burning pain (Ars., Carb-ac., Lach.).

Malignant pustules; *black or blue blisters*; often fatal in twenty-four or forty-eight hours (Lach., Pyrog.).

Carbuncle; *with horrible burning pains*; discharge of ichorous offensive pus.

Dissecting wounds especially if tendency is to become gangrenous; septic fever, marked prostration (Ars., Pyrog.).

Suspicious insect stings. If the swelling changes color and red streaks from the wound map out the course of lymphatics (Lach., Pyrog.).

Septic inflammation from absorption of pus or other deleterious substances, with burning pain and great prostration (Ars., Pyrog.).

Epidemic spleen diseases of cattle, horses and sheep.

Bad effects from inhaling foul odor of putrid fever or dissecting wound poisoning by foul breath (Pyrog.).

Hering says: "To call a carbuncle a surgical disease is the greatest absurdity. An incision is always injurious and often fatal. A case has never been lost under the right kind of treatment, and it should always be treated by internal medicine only."

Relationship

Similar: To, Ars., Carb-ac., Lach., Sec., Pyrog., in malignant and septic conditions.

Compare: Euph. in the terrible pains of cancer, carbuncle or erysipelas when Ars. or Anthraci. fail to >.

ANTIMONIUM CRUDUM

Sulphide of Antimony SbS_3

For children and young people *inclined to grow fat* (Calc.); for the extremes of life.

Old people with morning diarrhea, suddenly become constipated, or alternate diarrhea and constipation; pulse hard and rapid.

ANTIMONIUM CRUDUM

Sensitive to the cold, < after taking cold.

Child is fretful, peevish, **cannot bear to be touched or looked at;** sulky; does not wish to speak or be spoken to (Ant-t., Iod., Sil.); angry at every little attention.

Great sadness, with weeping.

Loathing life.

Anxious, lachrymose mood, the slightest thing affects her (Puls.); abject despair, suicide by drowning.

Irresistible desire to talk in rhymes or repeat verses.

Sentimental mood in the moonlight, especially ecstatic love; bad effects of disappointed affection (Calc-p.).

Nostrils and labial commissures sore, cracked and crusty.

Headache: After river bathing; from taking cold; alcoholic drinks; deranged digestion, acids; fat, fruit; suppressed eruption.

Gastric complaints from *over-eating;* stomach weak, digestion easily disturbed; **a thick milky-white coating on the tongue,** which is the red strand of the remedy; very subject to canker sores in the mouth (Arg-n., Sulph.).

Longing for acids and pickles.

Gastric and intestinal affections; from bread and pastry; acids, especially vinegar; sour or bad wine; after cold bathing; over-heating; hot weather.

Constant discharge of flatus, up and down, for years; belching, tasting of ingesta.

ANTIMONIUM CRUDUM

Mucus: In large quantities from posterior nares by hawking; from anus, *ichorous, oozing,* staining yellow; *mucus piles.*

Disposition to abnormal growths of the skin; fingernails do not grow rapidly; crushed nails grow in splits like warts with horny spots.

Large horny corns on soles of feet (Ran-b.); *very sensitive when walking,* especially on stone pavements.

Loss of voice from becoming over-heated.

Cannot bear *the heat of sun;* worse from over-exertion in the sun (Lach., Nat-m.) ; < from over-heating near the fire; *exhausted in warm weather;* ailments from sunburn.

Whooping cough: < by being over-heated in the sun or in a warm room; from cold washing.

When symptoms reappear they change locality or go from one side of the body to the other.

Aversion to cold bathing; child cries when washed or bathed with cold water; cold bathing causes violent headache; causes suppressed menses; colds from swimming or falling into the water (Rhus-t.).

Relationship

Complementary: Squilla.

Similar: To , Bry., Ip., Lyc., Puls., in gastric complaints.

Follows well: After, Ant-c., Puls., Merc., Sulph.

Aggravation

After eating; cold baths; acids or sour wine; *after heat of sun or fire;* extremes of cold, or heat.

Amelioration

In the open air; during rest; after a warm bath.

ANTIMONIUM TARTARICUM

Tartar Emetic

Adapted to torpid, phlegmatic persons; the hydrogenoid constitution (of Grauvogl).

Diseases originating from exposure in damp basements or cellars (Ars., Aran., Ter.).

Through the pneumogastric nerve it depresses the respiration and circulation, thus producing the keynote of the remedy, viz., *when the patient coughs there appears to be a large collection of mucus in the bronchi;* it seems as if much would be expectorated, but nothing comes up.

Child clings to those around; wants to be carried; cries and whines if anyone touches it; will not let you feel the pulse (Ant-c., Sanic.).

Face cold, blue, pale, covered with cold sweat (Tab.).

Tongue coated, pasty, thick, white, with reddened papillae and red edges; red in streaks; very red, dry in the middle; *extraordinary craving for apples* (Aloe; for acids, pickles, Ant-c.).

Vomiting: In any position except lying on right side; until he faints; followed by *drowsiness and prostration;* of cholera morbus with diarrhea and cold sweat, a dose after each attack (Verat.).

Asphyxia: Mechanical, as apparent death from drowning; from mucus in bronchi; from impending paralysis of lungs; from foreign bodies in larynx or trachea; with *drowsiness and coma.*

Great sleepiness or irresistible inclination to sleep, with nearly all complaints (Nux-m., Op.).

Child at birth pale, breathless, gasping; asphyxia neonatorum. Relieves the "death-rattle" (Tarent.).

Icterus with pneumonia, especially of right lung.

Relationship

Similar: To, Lycopodium, but spasmodic motion of alae is replaced by dilated nostrils; to Veratrum, both have diarrhea, colic, vomiting, coldness and craving for acids; to Ipecacuanha, but more drowsiness from defective respiration, nausea, but > after vomiting.

When lungs seem to fail, patient becomes sleepy, cough declines or ceases, it supplants Ip.

For bad effects of vaccination when Thuja fails and Silicea is not indicated.

Before Silicea in dyspnea from foreign bodies in the larynx or trachea; Puls. in suppressed gonorrhea; Ter. from damp basements.

Children not esily impressed when Ant-t. seems indicated in coughs, require Hepar.

In spring and autumn, when damp weather commences, cough of children gets worse.

Aggravation

In damp, cold weather; lying down at night; warmth of room; change of weather in spring (Kali-s., Nat-s.),

Amelioration

Cold open air; sitting upright; expectorating; lying on right side (Tab.).

APIS MELLIFICA

Poison of the Honey Bee *Apium Virus*

Adapted to the strumous constitution; glands enlarged, indurated; scirrhus or open cancer.

Women, especially widows; children and girls who, though generally careful, become awkward, and let things fall while handling them (Bov.).

Bad effects of acute exanthema imperfectly developed or suppressed (Zinc.); measles, scarlatina, urticaria.

Ailments from jealousy, fright, rage, vexation, bad news.

Irritable; nervous; fidgety; hard to please.

Weeping disposition; cannot help crying; discouraged, despondent (Puls.).

APIS MELLIFICA

Sudden, shrill, piercing screams from children while waking or sleeping (Helle.).

Edema; bag-like, puffy swelling *under the eyes* (over the eyes, Kali-c.); of the hands and feet, dropsy, without thirst (with thirst, Acet-ac., Apoc.).

Extreme sensitiveness to touch (Bell., Lach.).

Pain: **Burning, stinging, sore;** suddenly migrating from one part to another (Kali-bi., Lac-c., Puls.).

Thirstlessness; in anasarca; ascites (Aceticum acidum, but face more waxy and great thirst).

Incontinence of urine, with great irritation of the parts; can scarcely retain the urine a moment, and when passed scalds severely; frequent, painful, scanty, bloody.

Constipation: Sensation in abdomen as if something tight would break if much effort were used.

Diarrhea: Of drunkards; in eruptive diseases, especially if eruption be suppressed; involuntary from every motion, as though *anus was wide open* (Phos.).

Affects right side; enlargement or dropsy of right ovary; right testicle.

Intermittent fever; chill 3 p.m, *with thirt,* always (Ign.); < warm room and from external heat (Thuj., 3 a.m. and at 3 p.m.).

Relationship

Complementary: Nat-m.

Disagrees, when used either before or after Rhus-t.

Ars. and Puls. follow Apis well.

Has cured scarlatina albuminuria after Canth., Dig., Hell., failed.

Aggravation

After sleeping (Lach.); closed, especially warmed and heated rooms are intolerable; from getting wet (Rhus-t.), but better from washing or moistening the part in cold water.

Amelioration

Open air; cold water or cold bathing; uncovering; pains by coughing, walking or changing position; when sitting erect.

APOCYNUM CANNABINUM

Indian Hemp   *Apocynaceae*

Excretions diminished, especially urine and sweat.

Dropsy of serous membranes; acute, inflammatory.

Dropsy: *With thirst* (Acet-ac.), water disagrees or is vomited (Ars.); most cases uncomplicated with organic diseases; after typhus, typhoid, scarlatina, cirrhosis; after abuse of quinine.

Acute hydrocephalus, with open sutures; stupor, sight of one eye lost; constant and voluntary motion of one arm and one leg (left arm and leg, Bry.); forehead projected.

Amenorrhea in young girls, with bloating or dropsical extension of abdomen and extrimities.

Metrorrhagia: Continued or paroxysmal flow; fluid or clotted; nause, vomiting, palpitation; pulse quick, feeble, when moved; vital depression, fainting, when raising head from pillow.

Cough, short and dry, or deep and loose, during pregnancy (Con.).

Relationship

Similar: To, Aceticum acidum, Apis (no thirst), Ars., Chin., Dig., in dropsical affections.

Blatta orientalis has cured bad cases of general dropsy, after Apis, Apoc., and Dig. failed.—Haynes.

ARGENTUM METALLICUM

The Metal   *Pure Silver*

Tall, thin, irritable persons.

Ailments from abuse of mercury.

Constitutional effects of onanism.

Affects the cartilages, tarsal, ears, nose, Eustachian; the structures entering into joints.

Seminal emissions: After onanism; almost every night; without erection; with atrophy of penis.

Crushed pain in the testicles (Rhod.).

Prolapsus; with pain in left ovary and back, extending forward and downward (right ovary, Pall.); climacteric hemorrhage.

Exhausting, fluent coryza with sneezing.

Hoarseness; of professional singers, public speakers (Alum., Arum-t.).

Total loss of voice with professional singes.

Throat and larynx feel raw or sore on swallowing or coughing.

Laughing excites cough (Dros., Phos., Stann.) and produces profuse mucus in larynx.

When reading aloud has to hem and hawk; cough with easy expectoration of gelatinous, visxid mucus, looking like boiled starch.

Great weaknes of the chest (Stann.); worse left side.

Alteration in timbre of voice with singers and public speakers (Arum-t.).

Raw spot over bifurcation of the trachea; worse when using voice, talking or singing.

Relationship

Follows well: After, Alum.

Similar: To, Stann. in cough excited by laughing.

Aggravation

Riding in a carriage (Cocc.); when touched or pressed upon; talking, singing, reading aloud.

ARGENTUM NITRICUM

Silver Nitrate AgO, NO_5

Acute or chronic diseases from unusual or long-continued mental exertion.

Always think of Argentum nit. on seeing withered, dried up, old-looking patients (thin, scrawny, Sec.).

Emaciation, progressing every year; most marked in lower extremities (Am-m.); marasmus.

Apprehension when ready for church or opera, **diarrhea sets in** (Gels.).

Time passes slowly (Cann-i.); impulsive, wants to do things in a hurry; must walk fast; is always hurried; anxious, irritable, nevous (Aur., Lil-t.).

Headache: Congestive, with fullness and heaviness; with *sense of expansion;* habitual gastric, of literary men; *from dancing;* hemicrania, pressive, screwing in frontal eminence of temple; ending in bilious vomiting; < from *any exhaustive mental labor;* > *by pressure or tight bandaging* (Apis, Puls.).

Acute granular conjunctivitis; *scarlet-red, like raw beef;* discharge profuse, muco-purulent.

Ophthalmia neonatorum: Profuse, purulent discharge; cornea opaque, ulcerated; lids sore, thick, swollen; agglutinated in morning (Apis, Merc., Rhus-t.).

Eye strain from sewing, < in warm room, > in open air (Nat-m., Ruta); diseases due to defective accommodation.

Craves sugar; child is fond of it, but diarrhea results from eating (craves salt or smoked meat, Calc-p.).

Belching accompanies most gastric ailments.

Flatulent dyspepsia: Belching after every meal; stomach, as if it would burst with wind; belching difficult, finally air rushes out with great violence.

Diarrhea; green mucus, *like chopped spinach in flakes;* turning green *after remaining on diaper; after drinking; after eating candy or sugar;* masses of mucolymph in shreddy strips or lumps (Asar.); with much noisy flatus (Aloe).

Diarrhea as soon as he drinks (Ars., Crot-t., Trom.).

Urine passes unconsciously day and night (Caust.).

Impotence; erection fails when coition is attempted (Agn., Calad., Sel.).

Coition: Painful in both sexes; followed by bleeding from vagina (Nit-ac.).

Metrorrhagia: In young widows; in sterility; with *nervous erethism at change of life* (Lach.).

Great longing for fresh air (Aml-ns., Puls., Sulph.).

Chronic laryngitis of singers; the high notes cause cough (Alum., Arg-met., Arum-t.).

Great weakness of lower extremities, with trembling; cannot walk with the eyes closed (Alum.).

Walks and stands unsteadily, especially when he thinks himself unobserved.

Convulsions preceded by great restlessness.

Sensation *of a splinter* in throat when swallowing (Dol., Hep., Nit-ac., Sil.); in or about uterus when walking or riding.

Chilly when uncovered, yet feels smothered if wrapped up; craves fresh air.

Relationship

Natrium mur. for the bad effects of cauterizing with nitrate of silver.

Coffea increases nervous headache.

Boys' complaints after using tobacco (Ars., Verat.).

Similar: To, Nat-m., Nit-ac., Lach., Aur., Cupr.

After Verat.; Lyc. follows well in flatulent dyspepsia.

Aggravation

Cold foods; cold air; eating sugar; ice cream; *unusual mental exertion.*

Amelioration

Open air; craves the wind blowing in his face; bathing with cold water.

The 200th or 1000th potency in watery solution as a topical application in ophthalmia neonatorum has relieved when the crude silver nitrate failed.

ARNICA MONTANA

Leopard's Bane   *Compositae*

Nervous women, sanguine plethoric persons, lively expression and very red face.

For the bad effects resulting from mechanical injuries; even if received years ago.

Especially adapted to those who remain long impressed by even slight mechanical injuries.

Sore, lame, bruised feeling all through the body, as if beaten; traumatic affections of muscles.

Mechanical injuries, especially with stupor from concussion; involuntary feces and urine.

After injuries with blunt instruments (Symph.).

Compound fractures and their profuse suppuration (Calend.).

Concussions and contusions, results of shock or injury; without laceration of soft parts; prevents suppuration and septic conditions and promotes absorption.

Nervous, cannot bear pain; whole body oversensitive (Cham., Coff., Ign.).

Everything on which he lies seems too hard; complains constantly of it and keeps moving from place to place in search of a soft spot (the parts rested upon feel sore and bruised, Bapt., Pyrog.; must move continually to obtain relief from the pain, Rhus-t.).

Heat of upper part of body; coldness of lower.

The face or head and face alone is hot, the body cool.

Unconsciousness: When spoken to answers correctly, but unconsciousness and delirium at once return (falls asleep in the midst of a sentence, Bapt.).

ARNICA MONTANA

Says there is nothing the matter with him.

Meningitis after mechanical or traumatic injuries; from falls, concussion of brain, etc. When suspecting exudation of blood, to facilitate absorption.

Hydrocephalus; *deathly coldness in forearm of children* (in diarrhea, Brom.).

Apoplexy: Loss of consciousness, involuntary evacuation from bowels and bladder; in acute attack, controls hemorrhage and aids absorption; should be repeted and allowed to act for days or weeks unless symptoms call for another remedy.

Conjunctival or retinal hemorrhage, with extravasation, from injuries or cough (Led., Nux-v.).

Gout and rheumatism, *with great fear of being touched or struck by persons coming near him.*

Cannot walk erect on account of a bruised sort of feeling in pelvic region.

Tendency to small, painful boils, one after another, extremely sore (small boils in crops, Sulph.).

Paralysis (left-sided); pulse full, strong; stertor, sighing, muttering.

Belching; eructations; foul, putrid, like rotten eggs.

Dysentery; with ischuria, fruitless urging; *long interval between the stools.*

Constipation: *Rectum loaded,* feces will not come away; ribbon-like stools from enlarged prostate or retroverted uterus.

Soreness of parts after labor; prevents post-partum hemorrhage and puerperal complications.

Retention or incontinence of urine after labor (Op.).

Relationship

Complementary: To, Acon., Hyper., Rhus-t.

Similar: To, *for soreness as if bruised*, Bapt., Chin., Phyt., Pyrog., Rhus-t., Staph.

Arnica follows well: After, Acon., Apis, Ham., Ip., Verat., is followed by Sul-ac.

In ailments from spirituous liquors or from charcoal vapors, Arn. is often indicated (Am-c., Bov.).

In spinal convulsions, compare with Hyper.

Aggravation

At rest; when lying down; from wine.

Amelioation

From contact; motion (Rhus-t., Ruta).

ARSENICUM ALBUM

White Oxide of Arsenic As_2O_3

Great prostration, *with rapid sinking of the vital forces;* fainting.

The disposition is:

(a) Depressing, melancholic, despairing, indifferent.

ARSENICUM ALBUM

(b) Anxious, fearful, restless, full of anguish.

(c) Irritable, sensitive, peevish, easily vexed.

The greater the suffering, the greater the anguish, restlessness and fear of death.

Mentally restless *but physically too weak to move;* cannot rest in any place; changing places continually; wants to be moved from one bed to another, and lies now here, now there.

Anxious fear of death; thinks it useless to take medicine, *is incurable,* is surely going to die; *dread of death* when alone, on going to bed.

Attacks of anxiety at night driving out of bed, < after midnight.

Burning pains; the affected parts burn like fire, as if hot coals were applied to parts (Anthraci.), **> by heat,** hot drinks, hot applications.

Burning thirst without special desire to drink; the stomach does not seem to tolerate, because it cannot assimilate, cold water; lies like a stone in the stomach. It is wanted, but he cannot or dare not drink it.

Cannot bear the smell or sight of food (Colch., Sep.).

Great thirst for cold water; *drinks often, but little at a time;* eats seldom, but much.

Gastric derangements; after cold fruits; ice cream; ice water; sour beer; bad sausage; alcoholic drinks; strong cheese.

Teething children are pale, weak, fretful, and want to be carried rapidly.

Diarrhea, *after eating or drinking;* stool scanty; dark-colored, offensive, and whether small or large, *followed by great prostration.*

Hemorrhoids: With stitching pain when walking or sitting, not at stool; preventing sitting or sleep; *burning pain < by heat;* fissures make voiding urine difficult.

Breathing, asthmatic; must sit or bend forward; springs out of bed at night, especially after twelve o'clock; *unable to lie down for fear of suffocation;* attacks like croup instead of the usual urticaria.

Rapid emaciation: With cold sweat and great debility (Tub., Verat.); of affected parts; marasmus.

Anasarca, skin pale, waxy, earth-colored (Acet-ac.).

Excessive exhaustion from least exertion.

Exhaustion is not felt by the patient while lying still; when he moves he is surprised to find himself so weak.

Symptoms generally worse from 1-2 p.m., 12-2 a.m.

Skin: Dry and scaly; cold, blue and wrinkled; with cold, clammy perspiration; like parchment; white and pasty; black vesicles and burning pain.

Bad effects from decayed food or animal matter, whether by inoculation, olfaction or ingestion.

Complaints return annually (Carb-v., Lach., Sulph., Thuj.).

Relationship

Complementary: All-s., Carb-v., Phos., Pyrog.

Ars. should be thought of in ailments from: *Chewing*

tobacco; alcoholism; sea bathing; sausage poisoning; dissecting wounds and anthrax poison; stings of venomous insects.

Aggravation

After midnight (1 to 2 a.m. or p.m.); *from cold; cold drinks or food;* when lying on affected side or with the head low.

Amelioration

From heat in general (reverse of Sec.) except headache, which is temporarily > by cold bathing (Spig.); burning pain > by heat.

ARUM TRIPHYLLUM

Indian Turnip   *Araceae*

Coryza; *acrid, fluent; nostrils raw.*

Nose feels stopped up inspite of the watery discharge (compare, Am-c., Samb., Sin-n.); sneezing < at night.

Acrid, ichorous discharge, excoriating inside of nose, alae, and upper lip (Ars., All-c.).

Constant picking at the nose until it bleeds; boring with the finger into the side of the nose.

Pick lips until they bleed; corners of mouth sore, cracked, bleeding (with malignant tendency, Cund.); bites nails until fingers bleed.

Patients pick and bore into the *raw bleeding surfaces* though very painful; scream with pain but keep up the boring (in diphtheria, scarlatina, typhoid).

Children refuse food and drink on account of soreness of mouth and throat (Merc.); are sleepless.

Saliva profuse, acrid, corrodes the mucous membrane; tongue and buccal cavity raw and bleeding.

Aphonia: Complete, after exposure to north-west winds (Acon., Hep.); from singing (Arg-n., Caust., Phos., Sel.).

Clergyman's sore throat; voice hoarse, uncertain, uncontrollable, changing continually; worse from talking, speaking or singing; orators, singers, actors.

Desquamation in large flakes; a second or third time, in scarlatina.

Typhoid scarlatina, with apathy, scanty or suppressed urine; threatened uremia.

The sore mouth and nose are guiding in malignant scarlatina and diphtheria.

Relationship

Useful: After Hep. and Nit-ac. in dry, hoarse, croupy cough; after Caust. and Hep. in morning hoarseness and deafness, and in scarlatina.

Should not be given low or repeated often, as bad effects often follow.

The higher potencies most prompt and effective.

ASARUM EUROPAEUM

European Snake Root   *Aristolochiaceae*

Nervous, anxious people; excitable or melancholy.

Imagines he is hovering in the air like a spirit (Lac-c.); lightness of all the limbs.

Cold "shivers" from any emotion.

Oversensitiveness of nerves, **scratching of linen or silk, crackling of paper is unbearable** (Ferr., Tarent.).

Sensation as if ears were plugged up with some foreign substance.

When reading, sensation in eyes as if they would be pressed asunder or outward; relieved *by bathing them in cold water.*

Cold air or cold water very pleasant to the eyes; sunshine, light and wind are intolerable.

Nausea; in attacks or constant (Ip.); < after eating, tongue clean (Sulph.); of pregnancy.

Unconquerable longing for alcohol; a popular remedy in Russia for drunkards.

"Horrible sensation" of pressing, digging in the stomach when waking in the morning (after a debauch).

Great faintness and constant yawning.

Relationship

Similar: To, Caust. in modalities; to Aloe, Arg-n., Merc., Podo., Puls., Sul-ac. in stringy, shreddy stools.

Aggravation

In cold and dry, or clear, fine weather (Caust.).

Amelioration

Washing face or bathing affected parts with cold water; in damp, wet weather (Caust.).

Followed: By, Bism., Caust., Puls., Sul-ac.

ASTERIAS RUBENS

Star-fish *Radiata*

For the sycotic diathesis; flabby, lymphatic; irritable temperament.

Easily excited by an emotion, especially by contradictions (Anac., Con.).

Heat of the head, as if surrounded by hot air.

Sanguinous congestion of the brain.

Apoplexy; face red, pulse hard, full, frequent.

Cancer of mammae; *acute lancinating pain;* drawing pain in breast; swollen, distended, as before the menses; breast feels drawn in.

A livid red spot appeared, broke and discharged; gradually invaded entire breast, very fetid odor; edges pale, elevated, mammilllary, hard, everted; bottom covered with reddish granulations.

Gait unsteady; muscles refuse to obey the will (Alum., Gels.).

Epilepsy; twitching over the whole body four or five days before the attack.

Constipation: Obstinate; ineffectual desire; stools of hard, round balls, like olives.

Diarrhea: Watery, brown, gushing out in a violent jet (Crot-t., Grat., Gamb., Jatr., Thuja.).

Sexual desire increased in women (Lil-t.).

Relationship

Similar: To, Murex, Sepia.

Compare: Carb-an., Con., Sil. in mammary cancer: Bell., Calc., Sulph. in epilepsy.

AURUM METALLICUM

Gold   *The Element*

Sanguine, ruddy people, with black hair and eyes; lively, restless, anxious about the future.

Old people; weak vision; corpulent; *tired of life.*

For constitutions broken down by bad effects of mercury and syphilis.

Pining boys; low-spirited, lifeless, weak memories, lacking in "boyish go"; testes undeveloped, mere pendent shreds.

Constantly dwelling on suicide (Naja; but is afraid to die, Nux-v.).

AURUM METALLICUM

Profound melancholy: Feels hateful and quarrelsome; desire to commit suicide; life is a constant burden; after abuse of mercury; with nearly all complaints.

Uneasy, hurried, great desire for mental and physical activity; cannot do things fast enough (Arg-n.).

Ailments from fright, anger, contradictions, mortification, vexation, dread, or reserved displeasure (Staph.).

Oversensitive; least contradiction excites wrath (Con.); to pain; to smell, taste, hearing, touch (Anac.).

Headache of people with dark olive-brown complexion; sad, gloomy, taciturn, disposed to constipation; from least mental exertion.

Falling of the hair, especially in syphilis and mercurial affections.

Hemiopia; sees only the lower half (sees only the left half, Lith-c., Lyc.).

Syphilitic and mercurial affections of the bones.

Caries: Of the nasal palatine and mastoid bones; ozena, otorrhea, excessively fetid discharge, pains worse at night; drive to despair; of mercurial or syphilitic origin (Asaf.).

Prolapsed and indurated uterus; from over-reaching or straining (Podo., Rhus-t.); from hypertrophy (Con.).

Menstrual and uterine affections, with great melancholy; < at menstrual period.

AURUM METALLICUM

Foul breath; in girls at puberty.

Sensation as if the heart stood still; as though it ceased to beat and then suddenly gave one hard thump (Sep.).

Violent palpitation; anxiety, with congestion of blood to head and chest after exertion; pulse small, feeble, rapid, irregular visible beating of carotid and temporal arteries (Bell., Glon.).

Fatty degeneration of heart (Phos.).

Relationship

Aurum follows, and is followed well by Syphilinum.

Similar: To, Asaf., Calc., Plat., Sep., Tarent., Ther., in bone, uterine disease.

Aggravation

In cold air; when getting cold; while lying down; mental exertion; many complaints come on only in winter.

Amelioration

In warm air, when growing warm, in the morning, and during summer.

BAPTISIA TINCTORIA

Wild Indigo   *Leguminosae*

For the lymphatic temperament.

Great prostration, with disposition to decomposition of fluids (Pyrog.); ulceration of mucous membranes.

All exhalations and discharges *fetid*, especially in typhoid or other acute disease; breath, stool, urine, perspiration, ulcers (Psor., Pyrog.).

Aversion to mental exertion; indisposed, or want of power to think.

Perfect indifference, dosen't care to do anything, inability to fix the mind on work.

Stupor; falls asleep while being spoken to or in the midst of his answer (when spoken to, answers correctly, but delirium returns at once, Arn.).

Tongue: At first coated white with red papillae; dry and yellow-brown in centre; later dry, cracked, ulcerated.

Face flushed, dusky, dark red, with a stupid, besotted, drunken expression (Gels.).

Can swallow liquids only (Bar-c.); least solid food gags (can swallow liquids only, but has aversion to them, Sil.).

Painless sore throat; tonsils, soft palate and parotids dark red, swollen; putrid, offensive discharge (Diph.).

Dysentery of old people; diarrhea of children, especially when very offensive (Carb-v., Podo., Psor.).

Cannot go to sleep because she cannot get herself together; head or body feels scattered about the bed. Tosses about to get the pieces together; thought she was three persons, could not keep them covered (Petr.).

In whatever position the patient lies, the parts rested upon feel sore and bruised (Pyrog.; compare, Arn., Pyrog.).

Decubitus in typhoid (Arn., Mur-ac., Pyrog.).

Relationship

Similar: To, Arn., Ars., Bry., Gels., in the early stages of fever with malaise, nervousness, flushed face, drowsiness, and muscular soreness.

When Ars. has been improperly given or too often repeated in typhoid of typhus.

After Baptisia: Crot-t., Ham., Nit-ac., and Ter. act well in hemorrhage of typhoid and typhus.

BARYTA CARBONICA

Barium Carbonate $BaCO_3$

Especially adapted to complaints of first and second childhood; the psoric or tubercular.

Memory deficient; forgetful, inattentive; child cannot be taught for it cannot remember; threatened idiocy.

Scrofulous, dwarfish children who do not grow (children who grow too rapidly, Calc.); scrofulous ophthalmia, cornea opaque; abdomen swollen; frequent attacks of colic; face bloated; general emaciation.

Children both physically and mentally weak.

Dwarfish, hysterical women and old maids with scanty menses; deficient heat, always cold and chilly.

Old, cachetic people; scrofulous, *especially when fat;* or those who suffer from gouty complaints (Fl-ac.).

Diseases of old men; hypertrophy or induration of prostate and testes; mental and physical weakness.

Apoplectic tendency in old people; complaints of old drunkards; headache of aged people, who are childish.

Persons subject to quinsy, take cold easily, even the least cold precipitates an attack of tonsillitis, prone to suppuration (Hep., Psor.).

Inability to swallow anything but liquids (Bapt., Sil.).

Hemorrhoids protrude every time he urinates (Mur-ac.).

Chronic cough in psoric children; enlarged tonsils or elongated uvula; < after slight cold (Alum.).

Swelling and indurations, or incipient suppuration of glands, especially cervical and inguinal.

Offensive foot sweat; toes and soles get sore; of the heels; throat affections *after checked foot sweat* (compare, Graph., Psor., Sanic., Sil.).

Great sensitiveness to cold (Calc., Kali-c., Psor.).

Relationship

Frequently useful before or after Psor., Sulph. and Tub.

After Bar-c., Psor. will often eradicate the al tendency to quinsy.

Similar: To, Alum., Calc-i., Dulc., Fl-ac., Iod., Sil.

Incompatible: After Calc. in scrofulous affections.

Aggravation

When thinking of his disease (Ox-ac.); lying on painful side; after meals; washing affected parts.

BELLADONNA

Deadly Nightshade   *Solanaceae*

Adapted to bilious, lymphatic, plethoric constitutions; persons who are lively and entertaining when well, but violent and often delirious when sick.

Women and children with light hair and blue eyes, fine complexion, delicate skin; sensitive, nervous, threatened with convulsions; tubercular patients.

Great liability to take cold; sensitive to drafts of air, especially when uncovering the head; from having the hair cut; tonsils become inflamed after riding in a cold wind (Acon., Hep., Rhus-t.; takes cold from exposure of feet, Con., Cupr., Sil.).

Quick sensation and motion; eyes snap and move quickly; pains come suddenly, last indefinitely and

BELLADONNA

cease suddenly (Mag-p.).

Pains usually in *short attacks;* **cause redness of face and eyes;** fulness of head and throbbing of carotids.

Imagines he sees ghosts, hideous faces, and various insects (Stram.); black animals, dogs, wolves.

Fear of imaginary things, wants to run away from them; hallucinations.

Violent delirium; disposition to bite, spit, strike and tear things; breaks into fits of laughter and gnashes the teeth; wants to bite and strike the attendants (Stram.); tries to escape (Hell.).

Head hot and painful; face flushed; eyes wild, staring, pupils dilated; pulse full and bounding, globular, like buckshot striking the finger; mucous membrane of mouth dry; stool tardy and urine suppressed; sleepy, but cannot sleep (Cham., Op.).

Convulsions during teething, with fever (without fever, Mag-p.); comes on suddenly, head hot, feet cold.

Rush of blood to head and face (Aml-ns., Glon., Meli.)

Headache, *congestive,* **with red face, throbbing of brain and carotids** (Meli.); < from slight noise, jar, motion, light, lying down, least exertion; > pressure, tight bandaging, wrapping up, during menses.

Boring the head into the pillow (Apis, Hell., Podo.).

Vertigo when stooping, or when rising after stooping (Bry.); on every change of position.

Abdomen tender, distended < by least jar, even of the bed; obliged to walk with great care for fear of a jar.

BELLADONNA

Pain in right ileo-caecal region, < by slightest touch, even of the bed cover.

The transverse colon protrudes like a pad.

Skin: Of a uniform, smooth, shining scarlet redness; dry, hot, burning; imparts a burning sensation to examining hand; the true Sydenham scarlet fever, where eruption is perfectly smooth and truly scarlet.

Pressing downwards as if the contents of abdomen would issue from the vulva; > standing and sitting erect; worse mornings (Lil., Mur-ac., Sep.).

Relationship

Complementary; Calcarea.

Belladonna is the acute of Calcarea, which is often required to complete a cure.

Similar: To, Acon., Bry., Cic., Gels., Glon., Hyos., Meli., Op., Stram.

Aggravation

From touch, motion, noise, draft of air, looking at bright shining objects (Lyss., Stram.); after 3 p.m., night, after midnight; while drinking; uncovering the head; summer sun; lying down.

Amelioration

Rest; standing or sitting erect; warm room.

BENZOICUM ACIDUM

$CH_6H_5CO.OH$

A gouty, rheumatic diathesis engrafted on a gonorrheal or syphilitic patient.

Gouty concretions; arthritis vaga; affects all the joints, especially the knee, cracking on motion; nodosities (Berb., Lith-c., Lyss.).

Urine dark brown, and the urinous odor highly intensified.

Enuresis nocturna of delicate children; dribbling urine of old men with enlarged prostate; strong characteristic odor; excess of uric acid.

Catarrh of bladder after suppressed gonorrhea.

Diarrhea of children; white, *very offensive*, exhausting liquid stools running "right through diaper" (Podo.); urine offensive and of a deep red color.

Cough; with expectoration of green mucus (Nat-s.); extreme weariness, lassitude.

Pains tearing, stitching, in large joints of big toe; redness and swelling of joints; gout < at night.

Relationship

Similar: To Cop., Kali-n., Ferr., Thuj., especially in enuresis after Kali-n. has failed; Berb., Lith-c. in arthritic complaints.

Useful after Colch. fails in gout; after abuse of Cop. in suppression of gonorrhea.

Incompatible: Wine, which aggravates urinary, gouty and rheumatic affections.

BERBERIS VULGARIS

Barberry   *Berberidaceae*

The renal or vesical symptoms predominate.

Pain in small of back; very sensitive to touch in renal region; < when sitting and lying, from jar, from fatigue.

Burning and soreness in region of kidneys.

Numbness, stiffness, lameness with painful pressure in renal and lumbar regions.

Pale, earthy complexion, with sunken cheeks and hollow, blue-encircled eyes.

Rheumatic and gouty complaints, with diseases of the urinary organs.

Colic from gall-stones.

Bilious colic, followed by jaundice; clay-colored stools; fistula in ano, with bilious symptoms and itching of the parts; short cough and chest complaints, especially after operations for fistulae (Calc-p., Sil.).

Stitching, cutting pain from left kidney following course of ureter into bladder and urethra (Tab.; right kidney, Lyc.).

Renal colic, < *left side* (Tab.; either side, with urging and strangury, Canth.).

Bubbling sensation in kidneys (Med.).

Urine: Greenish, blood-red, with thick, slimy mucus; transparent, reddish or jelly-like sediment.

Movement brings on or increases urinary complaints.

Relationship

Similar: To, Canth., Lyc., Sars., Tab., in renal colic.

Acts well: After, Arn., Bry., Kali-bi., Rhus-t., Sulph., in rheumatic affections.

Aggravation

Motion, walking or carriage riding; any sudden jarring movement.

BISMUTHUM

Hydrated Oxide of Bismuth $Bi_{12}O_3OH_2$

Solitude is unbearable: desires company, child holds on to its mother's hand for company (Kali-c., Lil-t., Lyc.).

Anguish; *he sits, then walks, then lies, never long in one place.*

Headache returning every winter; alternating with, or attended by gastralgia.

Face, deathly pale, blue rings around the eyes. Toothache > by holding cold water in mouth (Bry., Coff., Puls.).

Vomiting: Of water as soon as it reaches the stomach, food retained longer (vomits food and water, Ars.); of *enormous quantities,* at intervals of several days when food has filled the stomach; of all fluids as soon as taken; and purging, offensive stools (watery stools, Verat.); *with convulsive gagging and inexpressible pain, after laparotomy* (Nux-v., Staph.).

Stomach: Pressure as from a load *in one spot;* alternating with burning; pain crampy, spasmodic; with irritation, cardialgia and pyrosis.

Cholera morbis and summer complaint, when *vomiting predominates;* stool foul; papescent, watery, offensive, very prostrating (Ars., Verat.).

BORAX

Biborate of Soda

Dread of downward motion in nearly all complaints.

Great anxiety from downward motion; when laying the child down on a couch or in the crib, cries and clings to the nurse; when rocking, dancing, swinging; *going down stairs, or rapidly down hill;* horse back-riding (compare, Sanic.).

Children awake suddenly, screaming and graping sides of cradle, without apparent cause (Apis, Cina, Stram.).

Excessively nervous, easily frightened by the slightest noise or an unusual sharp sound, a cough, sneeze, a cry, lighting a match, etc. (Asar., Calad.).

Hair becomes frowsy and tangled; splits, sticks together at the tips; if these bunches are cut off, they form again, cannot be combed smooth (Fl-ac., Lyc., Psor., Tub.).

Eyelashes: Loaded with dry, gummy exudation; agglutinated in morning; turn inward and inflame the eye, especially at outer canthus; tendency to "wild hairs."

Nostrils crusty, inflamed; tip of nose shining red; *red noses of young women.*

Stoppage of right nostril, or first right then left with constant blowing of nose (Am-c., Lac-c., Mag-m.).

Aphthae: In the mouth, on the tongue, inside of the cheek; easily bleeding when eating or touched; prevents child from nursing; with hot mouth, dryness and thirst (Ars.); cracked and bleeding tongue (Arum); salivation, especially during dentition.

Aphthous sore mouth; is wore from touch; eating salty or sour food; of old people, often from plate of teeth (Alumn.).

Child has frequent urination and screams before urine passes (Lyss., Sanic., Sars.).

Leucorrhea: Profuse, albuminous, starchy with sensation as if warm water were flowing down; for two weeks between the catamenia (compare, Bov., Con.).

Skin: Unhealthy, slight injuries suppurate (Calen., Hep., Merc., Sil.).

Relationship

Borax follows: Calc., Psor., Sanic., Sulph.

Is followed: By, Ars., Bry., Lyc., Phos., Sil.

Incompatible: Should not be used before or after, Aceticum acidum, vinegar, wine.

Aggravation

Downward motion; from sudden slight noises; smoking, which may bring on diarrhea; damp, cold weather; before urinating.

Amelioration

Pressure; holding painful side with hand.

BOVISTA

Puffball *Fungi*

Persons who suffer from tettery eruptions, dry or moist.

Adapted to old maids with palpitation.

Stammering children (Stram.).

Discharge from nose and all mucous membranes *very tough, stringy, tenacious* (Kali-bi.).

Usually deep impression on finger, from using blunt instruments, scissors, knife, etc.

Intolerance of tight clothing around the waist (Calc., Lach., Sulph.).

Sweat in axilla, smells like onion.

Hemorrhage: After extraction of teeth (Ham.); from wounds; epistaxis.

Great weakness of joints and weariness of hands and feet.

Awkwardness, inclined to drop things from hands (Apis); objects fall from powerless hands.

Menses: Flow *only at night*, not in the daytime (Mag-c.; only during day, ceases lying, Cact., Caust., Lil-t.); diarrhea before and during menses (Am-c.); occasional show every few days between periods (Borx.); every two weeks dark and clotted; with painful bearing down (Sep.).

Intolerable itching at tip of coccyx, must scratch till parts become raw and sore.

Relationship

Compare: Am-c., Bell., Calc., Mag-s., Sep. in menstrual irregularities.

Bovista antidotes, effects of local applications of tar; suffocation from gas.

When Rhus-t. seems indicated but fails to cure, in chronic urticaria.

BROMIUM

Bromine   *The Element*

It acts best, but not exclusively, on persons with *light blue eyes, flaxen hair, light eyebrows, fair, delicate skin; blonde, red-cheeked, scrofulous girls.*

Sensation of cobweb on the face (Bar-c., Borx., Graph.).

Fan-like motion of alae nasi (Ant-t., Lyc.).

Sailors suffer from asthma "on shore".

Stony, hard, scrofulous or tuberculous swelling of glands, especially on lower jaw and throat (thyroid, submaxillary, parotid, testes).

Diphtheria: Where the membrane forms in pharynx; beginning in bronchi, trachea or larynx, and extending upwards; *chest pains running upwards.*

Membranous and diphtheritic croup; *much rattling of mucus during cough,* but no choking (as in Hepar); sounds loose, but no expectoration (Ant-t.).

Croupy symptoms with hoarseness during whooping cough; gasping for breath.

Dyspnea: Cannot inspire deep enough; as if breathing through a sponge or the air passages were full of smoke or vapor of sulphur; rattling, sawing; voice inaudible; danger of suffocation from mucus in larynx (in bronchi, Ant-t.).

Hypertrophy of heart from gymnastics in growing boys (from calisthenics in young girls, Caust.).

Physometra; loud emission of flatus from the vagina (Lyc.); membranous dysmenorrhea (Lac-c.).

Cold sensation in larynx on inspiration (Rhus-t., Sulph.); > after shaving (< after shaving, Carb-an.).

Relationship

Compare: In croup and croupy affections, Chlor., Hep., Iod., Spong.

Hard goitre cured after Iod. failed.

Brom. has cured in croup after failure of Iod., Phos., Hep., Spong., especially in relapses after Iod.

"The chief distinction between Brom. and Iod. is, the former cures the blue-eyed and the latter the black-eyed patients." — Hering.

BRYONIA ALBA

White Bryony, Wild Hop *Cucurbitaceae*

It is best adapted to persons of a gouty or rheumatic diathesis; prone to so-called *bilious attacks.*

Bryonia patients are irritable, inclined to be vehement and angry; dark or black hair, dark complexion, firm muscular fibre; dry, nervous, slender people (Nux-v.).

Pains: Stitching, tearing, worse at night; < **by motion,** *inspiration, coughing;* > **by absolute rest, and lying on painful side** (Ptel., Puls.; stitching pain, but < and > are opposite, Kali-c.).

Excessive dryness of mucous membranes of entire body; lips and tongue dry, parched, cracked; stool, dry as if burnt; cough *dry, hard, racking,* with scanty expectoration; urine, dark and scanty; **great thirst.**

Vicarious menstruation; *nosebleed when menses should appear* (Phos.); blood spitting, or hemoptysis.

Ailments from chagrin, mortification, *anger* (Coloc.,

BRYONIA ALBA

Staph.); violence, with chilliness and coldness; *after anger chilly,* but with head hot and face red (Aur.).

Complaints: When warm weather sets in, after cold days; from cold drinks or ice in hot weather; *after taking cold or getting hot in summer;* from chilling when overheated; kicks the covers off; from exposure to draft, cold wind (Acon., Hep.); suppressed discharges, of menses, milk or eruption of acute exanthema.

One of the chief characteristics of Bryonia is **aggravation from any motion,** and corresponding relief from **absolute rest, either mental or physical.**

Desires things immediately which are not to be had, or which when offered are refused.

Children dislike to be carried, or to be raised.

Delirium: Talks constantly about his business; desire to get out of bed and go home (Cimic., Hyos.).

Constant motion of left arm and leg (Apoc., Hell.).

Patient cannot sit up from nausea and faintness.

Great thirst for *large quantities at long intervals.*

Headache: When stooping, as if brain would burst through forehead; *from ironing* (Sep.); on coughing; in morning after rising or when first opening the eyes; commencing in the morning, gradually increasing until evening; from constipation (Aloe, Coll., Op.).

Pressure as from stone at pit of the stomach; relieved by eructation (Nux-v., Puls.).

Constipation: *Inactive, no inclination; stool large, hard, dark, dry, as if burnt;* on going to sea (Plat.).

Diarrhea: During a spell of hot weather; bilious, acrid with soreness of anus; like dirty water; of undigested food; from cold drinks when overheated, from fruit or sour krout; < *in morning, on moving*, even a hand or foot.

Mammae heavy, of a stony hardness; pale but hard; hot and painful; **must support the breast** (Phyt.).

Cough: Dry, spasmodic, *with gagging and vomiting* (Kali-c.); with stitches in side of chest; with headache as if head would fly to pieces; < after eating, drinking, entering *a warm room*, a deep inspiration.

Relationship

Complementary: Alumina, Rhus tox.

Similar: To, Bell., Hep. for hasty speech and hasty drinking.

To Ran-b. in pleuritic or rheumatic pains in chest.

To Ptel. aching heaviness in hepatic region; > lying on right side, *greatly < lying on left side;* turning to the left causes a dragging sensation.

After Bryonia: Alum., Kali-c., Nux-v., Phos., Rhus-t., Sulph.

Aggravation

Motion, exertion, *touch;* cannot sit up, gets faint or sick or both; warmth, warm fold; suppressed discharges of any kind.

Amelioration

Lying, especially *on painful side* (Ptel., Puls.); pressure; rest; cold, eating cold things.

CACTUS GRANDIFLORUS

Night-blooming Cereus *Cactaceae*

Sanguinous congestions in persons of plethoric habit (Acon.); often resulting in hemorrhage; sanguinous apoplexy.

Fear of death; believes the disease incurable (Ars.).

Hemorrhage: From nose, lungs, stomach, rectum, bladder (Crot-t., Mill., Phos.).

Headache, pressing like a heavy weight on vertex (> by pressure, Meny.); climacteric (Glon., Lach.).

Headache and neuralgia; congestive, periodic, right-sided; severe, throbbing, pulsating pain.

Whole body feels as if caged, *each wire being twisted tighter and tighter.*

Constriction: Of throat, chest, heart, bladder, rectum, uterus, vagina; often caused or brought on by the slightest contact.

Oppression of chest, as from a great weight; as if an iron band prevented normal motion.

Sensation of a cord tightly tied around lower part of chest, marking attachment of diaphragm.

Heart feels as if clasped and unclasped rapidly by **an iron hand;** as if bound, "had no room to beat."

Pains everywhere; darting, springing like chain lightning, and ending with a sharp, vice-like grip, only to be again renewed.

Menstrual flow ceases when lying down (Bov., Caust.).

Palpitation: Day and night; worse when walking and lying on left side (Lach.); at approach of menses.

Fever paroxysm returns at 11 a.m. and 11 p.m.

Relationship

Compare: Acon., Dig., Gels., Kalm., Lach., Tab.

CALADIUM

American Arum   *Araceae*

Very sensitive to noise; slightest noise startles from sleep (Asar., Nux-v., Tarent.).

Eructations, frequent, of very little wind, as if stomach were full of dry food.

Impotence: With mental depression; *relaxed penis, with sexual desire and excitement* (Lyc., Sel.).

No erections, even after caress; no emission, no orgasm during an embrace (Calc., Sel.).

Pruritus vaginae; induces onanism (Orig., Zinc.); during pregnancy; with mucus discharge.

Falls asleep during evening fever and wakes when it stops.

Sweet sweat attracts the flies.

Mosquito and insect bites burn and itch intensely.

Aversion to motion; dreads to move (Bry.).

Destroys craving for tobacco.

CALCAREA ARSENICOSA

Arsenite of Lime

Great mental depression.

The slightest emotion causes palpitation of heart (Lith-c.).

Rush of blood to head and left chest (Aml-ns., Glon.).

Epilepsies, from valvular diseases of the heart.

Complaints of drunkards, after abstaining; craving for alcohol (Asar., Sul-ac.).

Complaints of fleshy women when approaching the menopause.

Relationship

Compare; Con., Glon., Lith-c., Puls., Nux-v.

Follows well: After, Conium, in lymphatic, psoric or tuberculous persons.

CALCAREA OSTREARUM

Middle Layer of Oyster Shell   *Calcium Carbonate*

Leucophlegmatic, blonde hair, light complexion, blue eyes, fair skin; tendency to obesity in youth.

Psoric constitutions; pale, weak, timid, easily tired when walking.

CALCAREA OSTREARUM

Disposed **to grow fat,** corpulent, unwieldy.

Children with red face, flabby muscles, who sweat easily and *take cold readily* in consequence.

Large heads and abdomens; fontanelles and sutures open; bones soft, develop very slowly.

Curvature of bones, especially spine and long bones; extremities crooked, deformed; bones irregularly developed.

Head sweats profusely while sleeping, wetting pillow far around (Sil., Sanic.).

Profuse perspiration, mostly on back of head and neck, or chest and upper part of body (Sil.).

Difficult and delayed dentition with characteristic head sweats, and open fontanelles.

During either sickness or convalescence, *great longing for eggs;* craves indigestible things (Alum.); aversion to meat.

Acidity of digestive tract; sour eructation, sour vomiting sour stool; sour odor of the whole body (Hep., Rheum).

Girls who are *fleshy, phethoric, and* **grow too rapidly.**

Menstruation *too early, too profuse, too long lasting;* with subsequent amenorrhea and chlorosis with menses scanty or suppressed.

Women: Menses too early, too profuse; feet habitually cold and damp, as if they had on *cold damp stockings;* continually cold in bed.

The least mental excitement causes profuse return of menstrual flow (Sulph., Tub.).

CALCAREA OSTREARUM

Fears she will lose her reason or that people will observe her mental confusion (Cimic.).

Lung disease of tall, slender, rapidly growing youth; upper third of right lung (Ars.; upper left, Myrt-c., Sulph.); oftener the guide to the al remedy than Phosphorus (compare, Tub.).

Diseases: Arising from *defective assimilation; imperfect ossification;* difficulty in learning to walk or stand; children have no disposition to walk and will not try; suppressed sweat.

Rawness of soles of feet from perspiration (Graph., Sanic.); blisters and offensive foot sweat.

Longing for fresh air (when in a room) which inspires, benefits, strengthens (Puls., Sulph.).

Coldness: General; *of single parts* (Kali-bi.); head, stomach, abdomen, feet and legs; aversion to cold open air, "goes right through her"; sensitive to cold, damp air; *great liability to take cold* (opposite of Sulph.).

Sweat: Of single parts; head, scalp wet, cold; nape of neck; chest, axille, sexual organs; hands, knees; feet (Sep.).

Pit of stomach swollen like *an inverted saucer,* and painful to pressure.

Uremic or other diseases brought on by standing on cold, damp pavements, or working while standing in cold water; modelers or workers in cold clay.

Feels better in every way when constipated.

Stool has to be removed mechanically (Aloe, Sanic., Sel., Sep., Sil.).

Painless hoarseness, < in the morning.

Desire to be magnetised (Phos.).

Relationship

Complementary: To, Bell., which is the acute of Calc.

Calcarea acts best: Before, Lyc., Nux-v., Phos., Sil.

It follows: Nit-ac., Puls., Sulph. (especially if pupils are dilated); is followed by, Kali-bi. in nasal catarrh.

According to Hahnemann, Calc. *must not be used before* Nit-ac. and Sulph.; may produce unnecessary complications.

In children it may be often repeated.

In aged people it should not be repeated; especially if the first dose benefited, it will usually do harm.

Aggravation

Cold air; wet weather; cold water; from washing (Ant-c.); morning; during full moon.

Amelioration

Dry weather; lying on painful side (Bry., Puls.).

CALCAREA PHOSPHORICA

Phosphate of Lime   *Calcium Phosphate*

For persons anemic and dark complexioned, dark hair and eyes; thin spare subjects, instead of fat.

CALCAREA PHOSPHORICA

During first and second dentition of scrofulous children; diarrhea and great flatulence.

Children: *Emaciated, unable to stand; slow in learning to walk* (Calc., Sil.); sunken, flabby abdomen.

Oozing of bloody fluid from navel of infants (of urine, Hyos.).

Rachitis: Cranial bones *thin and brittle;* **fontanelles and sutures remain open too long,** *or close and re-open;* delayed or complicated teething.

Spine weak; disposed to curvatures, especially to the left; unable to support body; neck weak, unable to support head (Abrot.).

Girls at puberty, tall, growing rapidly; tendency of bones to soften or spine to curve (Ther.).

At puberty: Acne in anemic girls with vertex headache and flatulent dyspepsia, > by eating.

Ailments from grief, disappointed love (Aur., Ign., Ph-ac.).

Feels complaints more when thinking about them (Helon., Ox-ac.).

Involuntary sighing (Ign.).

Non-union of bones; promotes callous (Symph.).

Rheumatism of cold weather; getting well in spring and returning in autumn.

Headache of school girls (Nat-m., Psor.); diarrhea.

At every attempt to eat, colicky pains in abdomen.

Fistula in ano, alternating with chest symptoms (Berb.); lack of animal heat; cold sweat and general coldness of body.

Relationship

Complementary: Ruta.

Similar: To, Carb-an., Calc-fl., Calc., Fl-ac., Kali-p.; to, Psor., in debility remaining after acute diseases; to, Sil., but sweat of head is wanting.

Acts best: Before Iod., Psor., Sanic., Sulph.; after Ars., Iod., Tub.

Aggravation

Exposure to damp, cold, changeable weather; east winds; *melting snow;* mental exertion.

Amelioration

In summer; warm dry, atmosphere.

CALENDULA

Marigold *Compositae*

Traumatic affections: To secure union by first intention and prevent suppuration.

In all cases of loss of soft parts when union cannot be effected by means of adhesive plaster.

External wounds with or without loss of substance; torn and jagged looking wounds; *post-surgical operations;* to promote healthy granulation and prevent excessive suppuration and disfiguring scars.

Traumatic and idiopathic neuroma (All-c.); neuritis from lacerated wounds (Hyper.); exhausted from *loss of blood and excessive pain.*

CALENDULA

Rupture of muscles of tendons; lacerations during labor; wounds penetrating articulations with loss os synovial fluids.

Wounds: With sudden pain during febrile heat; conbstitutional tendency to erysipelas (Psor.); old, neglected, offensive; threatening gangrene (Sal-ac.).

Ulcers: Irritable, inflamed, sloughing, varicose; *painful as if beaten* (Arn.); *excessive secretion of pus.*

Calendula is almost specific for clean, surgical cuts or lacerated wounds, to prevent excessive suppuration.

Relationship

Complementary: Hep., Sal-ac.

Similar: To, Hyper. in injuries to parts rich in sentient nerves where pain is excessive and out of all proportion to injury.

Similar: To, Arn. in traumatism without laceration of soft tissue.

Symph., Calc-p., for non-union of bones.

Sal-ac., prevents excessive suppuration; gangrene.

Sul-ac. in painful, gangrenous wounds; said to destroy septic germs.

Acts as well in potency as in tincture, applied locally, and may be administered internally at the same time.

CAMPHORA OFFICINALIS

Camphor *Lauraceae*

Pain better while thinking of it (Hell.; worse, Calc-p., Helon., Ox-ac.).

Persons physically and mentally weak and irritable. Exceedingly sensitive to cold air (Hep., Kali-m., Psor.).

Bad effects of shock from injury; surface of body, *cold, face pale, blue, tips livid;* **profound prostration.**

Surface **cold to the touch, yet cannot bear to be covered;** *throws off all coverings* (Med., Sec.).

Entire body painfully sensitive to slightest touch.

Tongue cold, flabby, trembling.

Sudden attacks of vomiting and diarrhea; *nose cold and pointed;* anxious and restless; *skin and breath cold* (Verat., Jatr.).

In first stages of cholera morbus and Asiatic cholera; severe, long-lasting chill (Verat.).

Great coldness of the surface with sudden and complete prostration of the vital force; often a remedy in congestive chill; pernicious intermittent (Verat.); pulse weak, externally small, scarcely perceptible.

Measles and scarlatina when eruption does not appear; with *pale or cold blue, hippocratic face;* child will not be covered (Sec.).

All sequelae of measles.

Relationship

Camphor antidotes nearly every vegetable medicine; also tobacco, fruits containing prussic acid, poisonous mushrooms; should not be allowed in the sick room in its crude form.

Compare: Carb-v., Op., Verat., Sec.

Amelioration

When *thinking of existing complaint;* warm air; drinking cold water.

Note for thought: All our progress as a school depends on the right view of the symptoms obtained by proving with Camphor and Opium. — Hering.

CANNABIS INDICA

Indian Hemp   *Urticaceae*

Very forgetful: Forgets his last words and ideas; *begins a sentence; forgets what he intends to speak;* inability to recall any thought or event on account of other thoughts crowding his brain (Anac., Lac-c.).

Constantly theorizing.

Laughs immoderately at every trifling word spoken to him.

Full of fun and mischief, then perhaps moaning and crying.

Great apprehension of approaching death.

Delirium tremens; excessive loquacity; exaggeration of time and distance.

Time seems too long (Arg-n.); a few seconds seem ages.

Distance seems immense; a few rods seem miles.

Sensation as if the calvarium was opening and shutting (Cimic.).

Sensation of swelling in the perineum or near the anus, as if sitting on a ball (with great quantities of ropy mucus in urine, Chin.).

Relationship

Compare: Bell., Hyos., Stram.

CANNABIS SATIVA

Hemp *Urticaceae*

Sensation as of *drops of water falling* on or from single parts; on the head, from the anus, stomach, heart.

Obstinate constipation, causing retention of the urine; constriction of anus.

Contraction of fingers after a sprain.

Dislocation of patella on going up stairs.

Dyspnea or asthma, where the patient can only breathe *by standing up*.

Choking in swallowing, things go down "the wrong way" (Anac.).

Acute, inflammatory stage of gonorrhea (second stage, burning after urination, discharge thick, yellow, pus-like, Cub.).

Urethra very sensitive to touch or pressure; cannot walk with legs close together, it hurts the urethra.

Pain extending from orifice of urethra backward, burning-biting, posteriorly more sticking, while urinating.

Tearing pains along urethra in a zigzag direction.

Relationship

Similar: To, Canth., Caps., Gels., Petros., in early stages of specific urethritis.

CANTHARIDES

Spanish Flies   *Cantharideae*

Over-sensitiveness of all parts.

Hemorrhages from nose, mouth, intestines, genital and urinary organs.

Pain; raw, sore, *burning in every part of body*, internally and externally; with extreme weakness.

Disgust for everything; drink, food, tobacco.

Drinking even small quantities of water increases pain in the bladder.

Constant urging to urinate, passing but a few drops at a time, which is mixed with blood (**sudden** desire to urinate and intense *itching* in urethra, Petros.).

Intolerable urging, before, during, and after urination; violent pains in bladder.

Burning, cutting pains in urethra during micturition; violent tenesmus and strangury.

Stool: Passage of white or pale; red, tough mucus, like *scrapings from the intestines,* with streaks of blood (Carb-an., Colch.).

Bloody, nocturnal emission (Led., Merc., Petr.).

Sexual desire; increased both sexes; preventing sleep; violent priapism, with excessive pain (Pic-ac.).

Tenacious mucus in the air passages (Bov., Kali-bi.); compare Cantharis if vesical symptoms correspond.

Skin: Vesicular erysipelas; vesicles all over body which are sore and suppurating.

Erythema from exposure to sun's rays (sunburn).

The burning pain and intolerable urging to urinate, is the red strand of Cantharis in all inflammatory affections.

Relationship

Similar: To, Apis, Ars., Equis., Merc.

Burns before blisters form and when they have formed. If the skin be unbroken, apply an alcoholic solution of any potency and cover with cotton; this will promptly relieve pain and often prevent vesication. If skin be broken use in boiled or distilled water, and in each case give potency internally.

CAPSICUM

Cayenne Pepper   *Solanaceae*

Persons with light hair, blue eyes, nervous but stout and plethoric habit.

Phlegmatic diathesis; lack of reactive force, especially with fat people, easily exhausted; *indolent, dreads any kind of exercise;* persons inclined to be jovial, yet get angry at trifles.

Children; *dread open air; always chilly;* refractory, *clumsy, fat, dirty,* and disinclined to work or think.

Desires to be let alone; wants to lie down and sleep.

Homesickness (of the indolent, melancholic), with *red cheeks* and sleeplessness.

Constriction: In fauces; throat; nares; chest; bladder; urethra; rectum.

Burning and smarting sensation, as from cayenne pepper, in throat and other parts, not > by heat.

Tonsillitis: With burning, smarting pain; intense soreness; *constriction of throat with* burning; inflamed, dark red, swollen.

The burning spasmodic constriction and other pains, **worse between acts of deglutition** (Ign.).

Painful swelling behind the ear (mastoid), extremely sore and sensitive to touch.

Every stool is followed by thirst and every drink by shuddering.

As the coldness of the body increases, so also does the ill-humor.

Nervous, spasmodic cough; in sudden paroxysms; as if head would fly to pieces.

With every explosive cough (and at no other time) there escapes a volume of pungent, fetid air.

Pain in *distant parts on coughing* (bladder, knees, legs, ears).

Relationship

Compare: Apis, Bell., Bry., Calad., Puls.

Cina follows well in intermittent fever.

The constricting, burning, smarting pains differentiate from Apis and Belladonna.

CARBO ANIMALIS

Animal Charcoal

Headache: As if a tornado in head; as if head had been blown to pieces; has to sit up at night and hold it together.

Diseases of elderly persons with marked venous plethora, blue cheeks, blue lips, and great debility.

Circulation feeble, stagnated, and vital heat sinks to a minimum; cynosis (Ant-t., Carb-v.).

Glands: Indurated, swollen, painful; in neck, axillae, groin, mammae; pains lancinating, cutting, burning (Con.).

CARBO ANIMALIS

Benign suppurations change into ichorous or malignant conditions.

Easily sprained from lifting, even small weights; straining and over-lifting easily produce great debility; ankles turn when walking.

Joints weak; easily sprained by slight exertion (Led.).

Aversion to open, dry, cold air.

After appearance of menses *so weak she can hardly speak* (Alum., Cocc.); menses flow only in morning.

Hearing confused; cannot tell from what direction a sound comes.

A stitching pain remaining in chest after recovery from pleurisy (Ran-b.).

Menstruation, leucorrhea, diarrhea are all exhausting (Ars.; all offensive, Psor.).

Relationship

Complementary: Calc., Phos.

Similar: To, Bad., Brom., Carb-v., Phos., Sep., Sulph.

Carbo animalis is often useful after bad effects from spoiled fish and decayed vegetables (Carb-v., All-c.).

Aggravation

After shaving (> after, Brom.); slightest touch; after midnight.

CARBO VEGETABILIS

Vegetable Charcoal

For the bad effects of exhausting diseases, whether in young or old (Chin., Phos., Psor.); cachectic persons whose vitality has become weakened or exhausted.

Persons who have never fully recovered from the exhausting effects of some previous illness; asthma dates from measles or pertussis of childhood; indigestion from a drunken debauch; bad effects of a long ago injury; has never recovered from effects of typhoid (Psor.).

Ailments: From quinine, especially suppressed intermitents; abuse of mercury, salt, salt meats; spoiled fish, meats or fats; *from getting overheated* (Ant-c.).

Bad effects from loss of vital fluids (Caust.); hemorrhage from any broken down conditions of mucous membranes (Chin., Phos.).

Weakness of memory and slowness of thought.

Epistaxis in daily attacks, for weeks, worse from exertion; face pale before as well as after a hemorrhage.

Hemorrhage from any mucus outlet; in systems broken down, debilitated; blood oozes from weakened tissues; vital force exhausted.

Hippocratic face; very pale, grayish-yellow, greenish, *cold with cold sweat;* after hemorrhage.

Looseness of teeth, easily bleeding gums.

CARBO VEGETABILIS

Patients crave things that make them sick; old topers crave whiskey or brandy; want clothing loose around abdomen.

Weak digestion; *simplest food disagrees;* excessive accumulation of gas in stomach and intestines < lying down; after eating or drinking, sensation as if stomach would burst; effects of a debauch, late suppers, rich food.

Eructations give temporary relief.

Diseases of the venous system predominate (Sulph.); symptoms of imperfect oxidation (Arg-n.).

Deficient capillary circulation causes blueness of skin and coldness of extremities; vital powers nearly exhausted; **desire to be constantly fanned.**

Hoarseness: < evenings; damp evening air; warm, wet weather; fails when exerted (< morning, Caust.).

Awakens often from cold limbs and suffers from *cold knees at night* (Apis).

Frequent, involuntary, cadaverous smelling stools, followed by burning; soft stool voided with difficulty (Alum.).

In the last stages of disease, with copious *cold sweat, cold breath, cold tongue, voice lost,* this remedy may save a life.

Relationship

Complementary: Kali-c.

Want of susceptibility to well-selected remedies (Op, Valer.).

Compare: Chin., Plb. in neglected pneumonia, especially in "old topers;" Ant-t. in threatened paralysis from inability to expectorate loosened mucus.

Opium: With lack of reaction after well-selected remedies fail to permanently improve (Valer.).

Phos. in easily bleeding ulcers.

Puls. bad effects from fat food and pastry.

Sulph., acrid smelling menstrual flow and erysipelas of mammae.

Aggravation

From butter, pork, fat food; abuse of quinine bark and mercury; from singing or reading aloud; in warm, damp weather.

Amelioration

From eructation; being fanned.

CARBOLICUM ACIDUM

Glacial Carbolic

The potencies are made with alcohol (an exception to the rule of preparing acids).

Pains are terrible; *come suddenly*, last a short time, disappear suddenly (Bell., Mag-p.).

Profound prostration, collapse; surface pale and bathed in cold sweat (Camph., Carb-v., Verat.).

Physical exertion, even much walking, brings on

abscess in some part, but generally in the right ear.—
R.T. Cooper.

Dull, heavy, frontal headache, as if *a rubber band were stretched tightly over the forehead,* from *temple to temple* (Gels., Plat., Sulph.).

When burns tend to ulceration and ichorous discharge.

Putrid discharges from mouth, nose, throat, nostrils, rectum; and vagina (Anthraci., Psor., Pyrog.).

Malignant scarlatina and variola (Am-c.).

Lacerated wounds from blunt instruments; bones bare, crushed; much sloughing of soft parts (Calen.).

Longing for whiskey and tobacco (Asar., Carb-v.).

Vomiting: Of drunkards, in pregnancy, sea-sickness, cancer; of dark, olive-green fluid (Pyrog.).

Dysentery: Fluid mucus, like scrapings of mucous membranes, and great tenesmus (Canth.); diarrhea, stool thin, involuntary, black, of an intolerable odor.

Constipation, with **horribly offensive breath** (Op., Psor.).

Leucorrhea: Acrid, copious, fetid, green.

Relationship

Compare: Ars., Kreos. in burns; ulcers with unhealthy, offensive discharges, Gels., Merc., Sulph.

Carbolic acid is antidoted by dilute cider vinegar, either externally or internally, when acid has been swallowed accidentally or taken for suicidal purposes.

CAULOPHYLLUM

Blue Cohosh *Berberidaceae*

Especially suited to women; ailments during pregnancy, parturition, lactation.

Rheumatism of women, especially of small joints (Act-sp.); erratic pains changing place every few minutes (Puls.); painful stiffness of affected joints.

Pains are intermittent, paroxysmal, spasmodic.

Chorea, hysteria or epilepsy at puberty, during establishment of menstrual function (Cimic.).

Leucorrhea: Acrid, exhausting; upper eyelids heavy, has to raise them with the fingers (Gels.); with "moth spots" on forehead (Sep.); *in little girls* (Calc.); preventing pregnancy.

Habitual abortion from uterine debility (Alet.; from anemia with profound melancholy, Helon.).

Spasmodic rigid os, delays labor; needle-like pricking pains in cervix.

Labor pains short, irregular, spasmodic; tormenting, useless pains in beginning of labor (Cimic.); no progress made. Will correct deranged vitality and produce efficient pains, if symptoms agree.

Hemorrhage, after hasty labor; want of tonicity; passive, after abortion (Sec., Thlas.).

After pains: After long exhausting labor; spasmodic, across lower abdomen; extend into groins (in the shins, Carb-v., Cocc.).

Lochia protracted; great atony; passive oozing for days from relaxed vessels (Sec.).

Relationship

Similar: To, Bell., Cimic., Lil-t., Puls., Sec., Thlas., Vib.

Similar to, labor pains of Puls., but mental condition opposite.

Similar to, Sep., "moth patches" and reflex symptoms from uterine irregularities.

CAUSTICUM

Hahnemann's Tinctura Acris Sine Kali

Adapted to persons with dark hair and rigid fibre; weakly, psoric, with *excessively yellow, sallow complexion;* subject to affections of respiratory and urinary tracts.

Children with dark hair and eyes, delicate, sensitive; skin prone to intertrigo during dentition (Lyc.), or convulsions with eruption of teeth (Stann.).

Disturbed functional activity of brain and spinal cord, from exhausting disease or severe mental shock resulting in paralysis.

Rawness or soreness: Of scalp, throat, respiratory tract, rectum, anus, urethra, vagina, uterus (as if bruised, Arn.; as if sprained, Rhus-t.).

Melancholy mood: Sad, hopeless; from care, grief,

sorrow; with weeping, "the least thing makes the child cry".

Intense sympathy for sufferings of others.

Ailments: From long-lasting grief and sorrow (Ph-ac.); from loss of sleep, night watching (Cocc., Ign.); from sudden emotions, fear, fright, joy (Coff., Gels.); from anger or vexation; from suppressed eruptions.

Children slow in learning to walk (Calc-p.).

Unsteady walking and easy falling of little children.

Constipation: Frequent, ineffectual desire (Nux-v.); stool passes better *when person is standing;* impeded by hemorrhoids; tough and shining, like grease; in children with nocturnal enuresis.

Urine involuntary: When coughing, sneezing, blowing the nose (Puls., Squil., Verat.).

Cough: With *rawness and soreness in chest;* with inability to expectorate, sputa must be swallowed (Arn., Kali-c.); relieved by drinking cold water; *on expiration* (Acon.); with pain in hips; remaining after pertussis; with expectoration chiefly at night.

Hoarseness with *rawness,* and aphonia < in the morning (< in the evening, Carb-v., Phos.).

At night, unable to get an easy position or lie still a moment (Eup-per., Rhus-t.).

Must move constantly but motion does not relieve.

Cannot cover too warmly, but warmth does not >.

Faint-like sinking of strength; weakness and trembling.

Cicatrices, especially burns, scalds, freshen up, become sore again; old injuries re-open; patients say "they never have been well since that burn."

Menses: Too early, too feeble; *only during the day*; cease on lying down.

Paralysis: **Of single parts;** vocal organs, tongue, eyelids, face, extremities, bladder; generally, of *right side*; form exposure to cold wind or draft; after typhoid, typhus or diphtheria; gradually appearing.

Drooping of upper eyelids; cannot keep them open (Caul., Gels., Graph.; of both lids, Sep.).

Rheumatic affections, with contraction of the flexors and stiffness of the joints; tension and shortening of muscles (Am-m., Cimx., Guaj., Nat-m.).

Warts: Large, jagged, often pedunculated; bleeding easily; exuding moisture; small, all over the body; on eyelids, face; on the nose.

Patient improves for a time, then comes to a "stand still" (Psor., Sulph.).

Relationship

Complementary: Carb-v., Petros.

Incompatible: Phos. Must not be used before or after Phos., always disagrees; the Acids; Coffea.

Compare: Arn., must swallow mucus; Gels., Graph., Sep. in ptosis; hoarseness, Rumx. and Carb-v. when < changes to evening; Sulph. in chronic aphonia.

Causticum antidotes paralysis from lead poisoning (bad effects of holding type in mouth of compositors), and abuse of Merc. or Sulph. in scabies.

It affects the right side most prominently.

Aggravation

In clear, fine weather; coming from the air into a warm room (Bry.); cold air, especially draft of cold air; on becoming cold; from getting wet or bathing.

Amelioration

In damp, wet weather; warm air.

CHAMOMILLA

Matricaria Chomomilla   *Campositae*

Persons, especially children, with light-brown hair, nervous, excitable temperament; oversensitive from use or abuse of coffee or narcotics.

Children, *new-born* and **during period of dentition.**

Peevish, irritable, oversensitive to pain, driven to despair (Coff.); snappish, cannot return a civil answer.

Child exceedingly *irritable, fretful*; **quiet only when carried;** impatient, wants this or that and becomes angry when refused, or when offered, petulantly rejects it (Bry., Cina, Kreos.); "too ugly to live"; cross, spiteful.

Piteous moaning of child because he cannot have what he wants; whining restlessness.

Patient cannot endure any one near him; is cross, cannot bear to be spoken to (Sil.); averse to talking, answers peevishly.

CHAMOMILLA

Complaint from anger, especially chill and fever.

Pain; seems unendurable, drives to despair; < by heat; < evening before midnight; with heat, thirst and fainting *with numbness of affected part*; eructations <.

One cheek red and hot, the other pale and cold.

Oversensitive to open air; great aversion to wind, especially about ears.

Toothache if anything warm is taken into the mouth (Bism., Bry., Coff.); on entering warm room; in bed; from coffee; during menses or pregnancy.

Labor pains: Spasmodic, distressing, wants to get away from them; tearing down the legs; press upward.

Diarrhea: From cold, *anger or chagrin;* **during dentition;** after tobacco; *in child-bed;* from downward motion (Borx., Sanic.).

Stool green, watery, corroding, like chopped eggs and spinach; *hot, very offensive, like rotten eggs.*

Nipples inflamed, tender to touch (Helon., Phyt.); infant's breasts tender to touch.

Milk runs out in nursing women (runs out after weaning, Con.).

Convulsions of children from nursing, *after a fit of anger in mother* (Nux-v. after fright in mother, Op.).

Violent rheumatic pains drive him out of bed at night, compel him to walk about (Rhus-t.).

Sleepy but cannot sleep (Bell., Caust., Op.).

Burning of soles at night, puts feet out of bed (Puls., Med., Sulph.).

Relationship

Complementary: Bell. in diseases of children, cranial nerves; Cham., abdominal nerves.

In cases spoiled by the use of opium or morphine in complaints of children.

Compare: Bell., Borx., Bry., Coff., Puls., Sulph.

Mental calmness contraindicates Chamomilla.

Aggravation

By heat; *anger*; evening before midnight; open air; in the wind; eructations.

Amelioration

From being carried; fasting; warm, wet weather.

CHELIDONIUM MAJUS

Celandine *Papaveraceae*

Persons of light complexion, blondes; thin, spare, irritable; subject to hepatic, gastric and abdominal complaints (Podo.); every age, sex and temperament.

Constant pain under the lower and inner angle of right scapula (Kali-c., Merc.; under the left, Chen-g., Sang.).

CHELIDONIUM MAJUS

Ailments: Brought on or renewed by change of weather (Merc.); all lessen after dinner.

Tongue coated thickly yellow, with red edges, showing imprint of teeth (Podo.; large, flabby, with imprint of teeth, Merc.).

Desire for *very hot drinks,* unless almost boiling, stomach will not retain them (Ars., Casc.).

Periodic orbital neuralgia (right side), with excessive lachrymation; *tears fairly gush out* (Rhus-t.).

Constipation: Stool, *hard, round balls* like sheep's dung (Op., Plb.); alternate constipation and diarrhea.

Diarrhea: At night; slimy, light-gray; bright-yellowish; brown or white, watery, pasty; involuntary.

Face, forehead, nose, cheeks remarkably yellow.

Yellow-gray color of the skin; wilted skin; of the palms of hands (Sep.).

Hepatic diseases; jaundice, pain in right shoulder.

Pneumonia of right lung, liver complications (Merc.).

Spasmodic cough; small lumps of mucus fly from mouth when coughing (Bad., Kali-c.).

Affects right side most; right eye, right lung, right hypochondrium and abdomen, right hip and leg; right foot cold as ice, left natural (Lyc.).

Old, putrid, spreading ulcers, with a history of liver disease, or of a tubercular diathesis.

Gall-stones, with pain under the right shoulder blade (terrible attacks of gall-stone colic, Card-m.).

Relationship

Chel. antidotes the abuse of Bry., especially in hepatic complaints.

Compare: Acon., Bry., Lyc., Merc., Nux-v., Sang., Sep., Sulph.

Ars., Lyc. and Sulph. follow well, and will often be required to complete the cure.

CICUTA VIROSA

Water Hemlock *Umbelliferae*

Women subject to epileptic and choreic convulsions; spasms of teething children, or from worms.

Convulsions; violent, *with frightful distortions* of limbs and whole body; with loss of consciousness of opisthotonos; renewed from slightest touch, noise or jar.

Puerperal convulsions: Frequent suspension of breathing for a few moments, as if dead; upper part of the body most affected; *continue after delivery*.

Epilepsy; with swelling of the stomach as from violent spasms of the diaphragm; screaming; red or bluish face; lockjaw, loss of consciousness and distortion of the limbs; frequent during the night; recurring, first at short, then at long intervals.

When reading, the letters seem to turn, go up or down or disappear (Cocc.).

During dentition, grinding of the teeth or gums; compression of the jaws as in lockjaw.

Abnormal appetite *for chalk and indigestible things;* for coal or charcoal; child eats them with apparent relish (Alum., Psor.).

Suffer violent shocks through head, stomach, arms, legs, which cause jerkings of the parts; head hot.

Injurious chronic effects from concussions of the brain and spine, especially spasms; trismus and tetanus from getting splinters into flesh (Hyper.).

Pustules which run together, forming thick, yellow scabs, on head and face. Sycosis menti.

Eczema: No itching; exudation forms into a hard lemon-colored crust.

Brain disease from suppressed eruptions.

Relationship

Compare: Hydr-ac., Hyper., Nux-v., Strych.

Aggravation

From tobacco smoke (Ign.); touch.

CINA MARITIMA

Worm Seed   *Compositae*

Adapted to children with dark hair, very cross, irritable, ill-humored, want to be carried, but carrying gives no relief; does not want to be touched; cannot bear anyone to come near it; averse to caresses; desires many things; but rejects everything offered (compare, Ant-t., Bry., Cham., Staph.).

Constantly digging and boring at the nose; picks the nose all the time; itching of nose; rubs nose on pillow, or shoulder of nurse (Teucr.).

Children, suffering from worms; pitiful weeping when awake, starts and screams during sleep; grinding of teeth (Cic., Spig.); ascarides (Teucr.).

Face is pale; sickly white and bluish appearance around mouth; sickly, with dark rings under the eyes; one cheek red, the other pale (Cham.).

Canine hunger: *Hungry soon after a full meal;* craving for sweets and different things; refuses mother's milk.

Urine: Turbid when passed, turns milky and semisolid after standing; white and turbid; involuntary.

Cough: Dry with sneezing; spasmodic, gagging in the morning; periodic, returning spring and fall.

Child is afraid to speak or move for fear of bringing on a paroxysm of coughing (Bry.).

Relationship

Compare: Ant-c., Ant-t., Bry., Cham., Kreos., Sil., Staph., in irritability of children.

In pertussis, after Drosera has relieved the severe symptoms.

Has cured aphonia from exposure when Acon., Phos., and Spong. had failed.

Is frequently to be thought of, in children, as an epidemic remedy, when adults require other drugs.

Santoninum sometimes cures worm affections when Cina seems indicated, but fails (Spig., Teucr.).

CINCHONA

Peruvian Bark　　　　　　　　　　　　*Rubiaceae*

For stout, swarthy persons; for systems, once robust, which have become debilitated, "broken down" from exhausting discharges (Carb-v.).

Apathetic, indifferent, taciturn (Ph-ac.); despondent, gloomy, has no desire to live, but lacks courage to commit suicide.

Ailments; from **loss of vital fluids, especially hemorrhages,** *excessive lactation, diarrhea, suppuration* (Chinin-s.); of malarial origin, with marked periodicity; return every other day.

After climacteric with profuse hemorrhages; acute diseases often result in dropsy.

Pains: Drawing or tearing; in every joint, all the bones. Periosteum, as if strained, sore all over; obliged to move limbs frequently, as motion gives relief; renewed by contact, and then gradually increase to a great height.

Headache: *As if the skull would burst;* intense throbbing of head and carotids, face flushed; from occiput over whole head; < sitting or lying, must stand or walk; after *hemorrhage or sexual excesses.*

Face pale, hippocratic; eyes sunken and surrounded by blue margins; pale, sickly expression as after excesses; toothache while nursing the child.

Excessive flatulence of stomach and bowels; fermentation, borborygmus; belching gives no relief

CINCHONA

(belching relieves, Carb-v.); < after eating fruit (Puls.).

Colic: At a certain hour each day; periodical, from gall-stones (Card-m.); worse at night and after eating; better bending double (Coloc.).

Great debility, trembling, aversion to exercise; **sensitive to touch,** *to pain, to drafts of air;* entire nervous system extremely sensitive.

Unrefreshing sleep or constant sopor; < after 3 a.m., wakens early.

Hemorrhages: of mouth, nose, bowels or uterus; *long continued;* longing for sour things.

Disposition to hemorrhage from every orifice of the body with ringing in ears, fainting, loss of sight, general coldness, sometimes convulsions (Ferr., Phos.).

Pains are < by slightest touch, but > by hard pressure (Caps., Plb.).

One hand icy cold, the other warm (Dig., Ip., Puls.).

Intermittent fever; paroxysm anticipates from two to three hours each attack (Chinin-s); returns every seven or fourteen days; *never at night;* sweat profusely all over on being covered, or during sleep (Con.).

Relationship

Complementary. Ferrum.

Follows well: Calc-p. in hydrocephloid.

Compare: Chinin-s. in intermittent fever, anticipating type.

Incompatible: After, Dig., Sel.

Is useful in bad effects from excessive tea drinking or abuse of chamomile tea, when hemorrhage results.

Aggravation

From *slightest touch; draft of air;* every other day; mental emotions; loss of vital fluids.

Amelioration

Hard pressure; bending double.

COCA

Erythroxylon Coca   ***Lineae***

For persons who are wearing out under the physical and mental strain of a busy life; who suffer from exhausted nerves and brain (compare, Fl-ac.).

Melancholy, from *nervous exhaustion; bashful,* timid, ill at ease in society.

Sad, irritable; delights in solitude and obscurity.

Longing for alcoholic liquors and tobacco; for the accustomed stimulants.

Want of breath; in those engaged in athletic sports; *shortness of breath* in old people; in those who use tobacco and whisky in excess.

Hemoptysis, with oppression of chest and dyspnea.

Sleepy, but can find no rest anywhere.

Violent palpitation: From incarcerated flatus (Arg-n., Nux-v.); from over-exertion; from heart strain (Arn., Borx., Caust.).

Bad effects: From mountain climbing or ballooning (Ars.); of stimulants, alcohol, tobacco.

Prevents caries of teeth.

Relationship

Compare: Patient desires light and company, Stram; desires darkness and solitude, Coca

Was first used as a tobacco antidote.

COCCULUS

Cocculus Indicus   *Menispermaceae*

For women and children with light hair and eyes, who suffer severely during menstruation and pregnancy; unmarried and childless women.

Adapted to book-worms; sensitive, romantic girls with irregular menstruation; rakes, onanists and persons debilitated by sexual excesses.

Nausea or vomiting **from riding in carriage, boat or railroad car** (Arn., Nux-m.), *or even looking at a boat in motion;* sea-sickness; car-sickness.

Headache: In nape and occiput; extending to the spine; as if highly bound by cord; with nausea, as if at sea; at each menstrual period; < lying on back of head.

Sick-headache from carriage, boat or train riding.

COCCULUS

Diseases peculiar to drunkards.

Loss of appetite, with metallic taste (Merc.).

Time passes too quickly (too slowly, Arg-n., Cann-i.).

Great lassitude of the whole body; it requires exertion to stand firmly; feels too weak to talk loudly.

Bad effects: From **loss of sleep,** *mental excitement and night watching;* feel weak if they lose but one hour's sleep; convulsions after loss of sleep; of anger and grief;

Trembling of arms and legs; from excitement, exertion or pain.

Vertigo, as if intoxicated upon rising in bed; or by motion of the carriage (Bry.).

Sensation: In abdomen of cutting and rubbing on every movement, as of sharp stones; of hollowness in head and other parts (Ign.).

During the effort to menstruate she is so weak she is *scarcely able to stand* from weakness of lower limbs (Alum., Carb-an.); after each period hemorrhoids.

Leucorrhea in place of menses, or between periods (Iod., Xan.); like the washings of meat; like serum, ichorous, bloody; during pregnancy.

Cannot bear contradiction; easily offended; every trifle makes him angry; speaks hastily (Anac.).

When fever assumes a slow "sneaking," nervous form, with vertigo; with disposition to anger.

Relationship

Compare: Ign. and Nux-v., in chorea and paralytic symptoms; Ant-t., in sweat of affected parts.

Has cured umbilical hernia with obstinate constipation, after Nux failed.

Aggravation

Eating, drinking, sleeping, smoking, talking; carriage riding, motion or swing of ship; rising up during pregnancy.

COFFEA CRUDA

Coffee   *Rubiaceae*

Tall, lean, stooping persons, dark complexion, sanguine choleric temperament.

Oversensitiveness; all the senses more acute, sight, hearing, smell, taste, touch (Bell., Cham., Op.).

Unusual activity of mind and body.

Full of ideas; quick to act, no sleep on this account.

Ailments: The bad effects of sudden emotions or pleasurable surprises (Caust.; exciting or bad news, Gels.); weeping from delight; alternate laughing and weeping.

Pains are felt intensely; seem almost insupportable, driving patient to despair (Acon., Cham.); tossing about in anguish.

Sleepless, wide-awake condition; impossible to close the eyes; physical excitement through mental exaltation (compare, Senecio, for sleeplessness from prolapsus, uterine irritation, during climacteric).

Headache: From over-mental exertion, thinking, talking; one-sided, as from a nail driven into the brain (Ign., Nux-v.); as if brain were torn or dashed to pieces; worse in open air.

Hasty eating and drinking (Bell., Hep.).

Toothache: Intermittent, jerking, relieved by holding ice-water in the mouth, but returns when water becomes warm (Bism., Bry., Puls., Caust., Sep., Nat-s.).

Relationship

Compare: Acon., Cham., Ign., Sulph.

Incompatible: Canth., Caust., Cocc., Ign.

Aggravation

Sudden mental emotion; *excessive joy;* cold, open air; narcotic medicines.

COLCHICUM AUTUMNALE

Meadow Saffron   *Liliaceae*

Adapted to the rheumatic, gouty diathesis; persons of robust vigorous constitution; diseases of old people.

External impressions, light, noise, strong odors, contact, bad manners, make him almost beside himself (Nux-v.); his sufferings seem intolerable.

Ailments: From grief or misdeeds of others (Staph.).

Pains are drawing, tearing, pressing; light or superficial during warm weather; affect the bones and deeper tissues, when air is cold; pains go from left to right (Lach.).

Smell painfully acute; nausea and faintness from the odor of cooking food, *especially fish,* eggs or fat meat (Ars., Sep.); bad effects from night watching (Cocc.).

Aversion to food; loathing even the sight or still more the smell of it.

The abdomen is immensely *distended with gas*, feeling as if it would burst

Burning, or icy coldness in stomach and abdomen.

Autumnal dysentery, discharges from bowels contain white shreddy particles in large quantities; white mucus; "scrapings of intestines" (Canth., Carb-ac.).

Urine: Dark, scanty or suppressed; in drops, with white sediment; bloody, brown, black, inky; contains clots of putrid decomposed blood, albumin, sugar.

Affected parts very sensitive to contact and motion.

Arthritic pains in joints; patient screams with pain on touching a joint or stubbing a toe.

Relationship

Compare: Bry. in rheumatic gout with serious effusions; in rheumatism in warm weather.

Often cures dropsy after Apis and Ars. fail.

Aggravation

Mental emotion or exhaustion; effects of hard study; *odor of cooking food.*

Motion; if the patient lies perfectly still, the disposition to vomit is less urgent. Every motion renews it (Bry.).

COLLINSONIA CANADENSIS

Stone Root *Labiatae*

Pelvic and portal congestion resulting in dysmenorrhea and hemorrhoids.

Congestion of pelvic viscera, with hemorrhoids, especially in latter months of pregnancy.

Dropsy from cardiac disease.

Palpitation; in patients subject to piles and indigestion; heart's action persistently rapid but weak.

After heart is relieved old piles reappear, or suppressed menses return.

Chronic, painful, bleeding piles; sensation as if sticks, sand or gravel had lodged in rectum (Aesc.).

Hemorrhoidal dysentery with tenesmus.

Alternate constipation and diarrhea; congestive inertia of lower bowel; stools sluggish and hard with pain and *great flatulence.* Constipation.

Pruritus in pregnancy with hemorrhoids, unable to lie down.

Relationship

In heart disease complicated with hemorrhoids

consult Collinsonia when Cact., Dig. and other remedies fail.

Has cured colic after Coloc. and Nux-v. had failed.

Compare: Aesc., Aloe, Cham., Nux-v., Sulph.

Aggravation

The slightest *mental emotion or excitement* aggravates the symptoms (Arg-n.).

COLOCYNTHIS

Squirting Cucumber　　　　　　　　*Cucurbitaceae*

Agonizing pain in abdomen **causing patient to bend double,** with restlessness, twisting and turning to obtain relief > by **hard pressure** (> by heat, Mag-p.).

Pain: Are worse after eating or drinking; compel patent to bend double (Mag-p.; < by bending double, Dios.); menses, suppressed by chagrin, colic pains.

Extremely irritable, impatient; becomes angry or offended on being questioned.

Irritable; throws things out of his hands.

Affections from anger, with indignation — colic, vomiting, diarrhea and suppression of menses (Cham., Staph.).

Vertigo: when quickly turning head, *especially to the left,* as if he would fall; from stimulants.

Sciatica: Crampy pain in hip, as though screws in a vise; lies upon affected side.

Shooting pain, like lightning shocks, down the whole limb, left hip, left thigh, left knee, into popliteal fossa.

Relationship

Complementary: Merc. in dysentery, with great tenesmus.

Compare: Gnaph. intense pain along right sciatic nerve, darting, cutting, from right hip joint down to foot; < lying down, motion, stepping; > by sitting.

Compare: With Staph. in ovarian or other diseases from bad effects of anger, reserved indignation or silent grief.

Aggravation

Anger and indignation; mortification caused by offense (Staph., Lyc.); cheese < colic.

Amelioration

From doubling up; hard pressure.

CONIUM MACULATUM

Poison Hemlock   *Umbelliferae*

The "Balm of Gilead" for diseases of old maids and women during and after climacteric.

Especially for diseases of old men; old maids; old bachelors; with rigid muscular fibre; persons with light hair who are easily excited; strong persons of sedentary habits.

Debility of old people; complaints caused by a blow or fall; cancerous and scrofulous persons with enlarged glands; rigid fibre.

No inclination for business or study; indolent, indifferent, takes no interest in anything.

Memory weak, unable to sustain any mental effort.

Morose; easily vexed; domineering, quarrelsome, scolds, will not bear contradiction (Aur.); excitement of any kind causes mental depression.

Dreads being alone, yet avoids society (Kali-c., Lyc.).

Glandular induration of stony hardness; of mammae and testicles in persons of cancerous tendency; after bruises and injuries of glands (compare, Aster.).

Breasts sore, hard and painful before and during menstruation (Lac-c., Kali-c.).

Vertigo: Especially **when lying down or turning in bed;** moving the head slightly, or even the eyes; must keep head perfectly still; in *turning the head to the left* (Coloc.); of old people; with ovarian and uterine complaints.

Cough: In spasmodic paroxysms caused by dry spot in larynx (in throat, Cimic.); with itching chest and throat (Iod.); worse at night, *when lying down,* and during pregnancy (Caust., Kali-br.).

Great difficulty in voiding urine; **flow intermits,** then flows again; prostatic or uterine affections.

Menses: *Feeble, suppressed; too late,* scanty, of short duration; with rash of small red pimples over body which ceases with the flow (Dulc.); stopped by taking cold; *by putting hands in cold water* (Lac-d.).

Leucorrhea; *ten days after menses* (Borx., Bov.); acrid; bloody; milky; profuse; thick; intermits.

Bad effects: Of **suppressed sexual desire,** or *suppressed menses;* non-gratification of sexual instinct, or from excessive indulgence.

Aversion to light without inflammation of eyes; worse from using eyes in artificial light; often the students' remedy for night work; intense photophobia (Psor.).

Sweat day and night, *as soon as one sleeps, or even when closing the eyes* (Chin.).

Relationship

Patients requiring Conium often improve from wine or stimulants; though persons susceptible to Conium cannot take alcoholic stimulants when in health.

Compare: Arn., Rhus-t., in contusions; Ars., Aster. in cancer; Calc., Psor. in glandular swellings.

Is followed well: By Psor., in tumors of mammae with threatening malignancy.

Aggravation

At night; lying down; turning or rising up, in bed; *celibacy.*

CROCUS SATIVUS

Saffron   *Iridaceae*

Frequent and extreme changes in sensations; *sudden, from the greatest hilarity to the deepest despondency* (Ign., Nux-m.).

Excessively happy, affectionate, wants to kiss everybody; the next moment in a rage.

Hemorrhage from any part, blood black, viscid, clotted, forming into **long black strings hanging from the bleeding surface** (Elaps).

Headache: During climacteric, throbbing, pulsating. < *during two or three days of accustomed menstrual flow;* nervous or menstrual headache before, during, or after flow (Lach., Lil-t., Sec.).

Eyes: Sensation, as if room were filled with smoke; as if had been weeping; as of cold wind blowing across the eyes; closing lids tightly gives >.

Nosebleed: **Black, tenacious, stringy, every drop can be turned into a thread;** with cold sweat in large drops on forehead (cold sweat, but wants to be fanned; with bright red blood, Carb-v.); in children who develop too rapidly (Calc., Phos.).

Dysmenorrhea; flow black; stringy, clotted (Ust.).

Sensation as if something alive were moving in the stomach, abdomen, uterus, arms or other parts of the body (Sab., Thuj., Sulph.); with nausea and faintness.

Chorea and hysteria with great hilarity, singing and

dancing (Tarent.); alternating with melancholy and rage.

Spasmodic contractions and twitchings of single sets of muscles (Agar., Ign., Zinc.).

Relationship

Nux-v., Puls., or Sulph. follow Crocus well in nearly all complaints.

Compare: In menstrual derangements (Ust.).

CROTALUS HORRIDUS

Poison of Rattlesnake   *Crotalidae*

Is indicated in strumous, debilitated, hemorrhagic, broken-down constitutions, during zymotic diseases; in inebriates; tendency to carbuncles or blood boils (Anthraci.).

Diseases caused by a previous low state of the system; low septic typhoid or malarial fever, chronic alcoholism, exhausted vital force; genuine collapse.

Apoplexy: Apoplectic convulsions in inebriates, hemorrhagic or broken down constitutions.

Hemorrhagic diathesis; blood flows from eyes, ears, nose, and every orifice of the body; *bloody sweat.*

Yellow color of conjunctiva; clears up vision after keratitis, or kerato-iritis.

Malignant jaundice; hematic rather than hepatic.

Purpura hemorrhagica; comes on suddenly from all orifices, skin, nails, gums.

Tongue fiery red, smooth and polished (Pyrog.); intensely swollen.

Malignant diphtheria or scarlatina; edema or gangrene of fauces or tonsils; pain < from empty swallowing; if vomiting or diarrhea come on.

Prostration of vital force; pulse scarcely felt; blood poisoning (Pyrog.).

Vomiting: Bilious, with anxiety and weak pulse; every month after menstruation; cannot lie on right side or back without instantly producing dark, green vomiting; black or coffee grounds, of yellow fever.

Diarrhea; stools black, thin, like coffee-grounds; offensive; from noxious effluvia or septic matters in food or drinks; from "high game" (Pyrog.); during yellow fever, cholera, typhoid, typhus.

Intestinal hemorrhage when occurring in typical septic or zymotic disease; blood dark, fluid, non-coagulable.

Dissecting wounds; insect stings; bad effects of vaccination.

Vicarious menstruation; in debilitated constitutions (Dig., Phos.).

Menopause; intense and drenching perspirations; faintness and sinking at stomach; prolonged metrorrhagia, dark, fluid, offensive; profound anemia.

Malignant diseases of uterus, great tendency to hemorrhage, blood dark, fluid, offensive.

Relationship

Compare: Elaps, Lach., Naja, Pyrog.

In Lach. skin cold clammy; Crot-h. cold and dry; Elaps, affections of right lung, expectoration of black blood.

CROTON TIGLIUM

Croton Oil Seeds　　　　　　　　*Euphorbiaceae*

Affects mucous membrane of intestinal tract, producing transudations of watery portions of blood, a copious, watery diarrhea (Verat.), and develops an acute eczema over whole body (Rhus-t.).

The bowels are moved as if by spasmodic jerks, "coming out like a shot" (Gamb.); *as soon as patient eats, drinks,* or even *while eating;* yellow watery stool.

Constant urging to stool followed by sudden evacuation, which is shot out of the rectum (Gamb., Grat., Podo., Thuj.).

Swashing sensation in intestines, as from water, before stool (rumbling before stool, Aloe).

Drawing pain through the chest from breast to scapula, of same side every time the child nurses; nipple very sore.

Intense itching of skin, but so tender is unable to scratch; > by gentle rubbing; eczema over whole body.

Intense itching of genitals of both sexes (Rhus-t.), vesicular eruption on male; so sensitive and sore is unable to scratch.

Cough; as soon as the head touches the pillow a spasmodic paroxysm of cough set in; suffocated, must walk about the room or sleep in a chair.

Relationship

Compare: Kali-br., Phos. in chronic infantile diarrhea; Sil. pain from nipple through to back when nursing.

Aggravation

Diarrhea; every motion; after drinking; while eating or nursing (Arg-n., Ars.); during summer; from fruit and sweetmeats (Gamb.); *the least food or drink.*

CUPRUM METALLICUM

Copper, Cu. *The Element*

Spasms and cramps: Symptoms disposed to appear periodically and in groups.

Mental and physical exhaustion from over-exertion of mind and *loss of sleep* (Cocc., Nux-v.); attacks of unconquerable anxiety.

A strong, sweetish, metallic, copper taste in the mouth with flow of saliva (Rhus-t.).

Constant prostration and retraction of the tongue, like a snake (Lach.).

While drinking, the fluid descends with a gurgling sound (Ars., Thuj.).

Cholera morbus or Asiatic cholera, with cramps in abdomen and calves of legs.

Bad effects of re-percussed eruptions (of non-developed, Zinc.), resulting in brain affections, spasms, convulsions, vomiting; of suppressed foot-sweat (Sil., Zinc.).

Convulsions, with blue face and clenched thumbs.

Cramps in the extremities; pains, soles, calves with great weariness of limbs.

Clonic spasms, *beginning in fingers and toes,* and spreading over entire body; during pregnancy; puerperal convulsions; after fright or vexation; from metastasis from other organs to brain (Zinc.).

Paralysis of tongue; imperfect, stammering speech.

Epilepsy: Aura begins in knees and ascends; < at night during sleep (Bufo); about new moon, at regular intervals (menses); from a fall or blow upon the head; from getting wet.

Cough has a *gurgling sound,* as if water was being poured from a bottle.

Cough, > by drinking cold water (Caust.; < by drinking cold water, Spong.).

Whooping cough: Long-lasting, *suffocating,* spasmodic cough; unable to speak; *breathless, blue face, rigid, stiff; three attacks* successively (Stann.); vomiting of solid food after regaining consciousness (Cann-i.); cataleptic spasm with each paroxysm.

After pains; severe, distressing, in calves and soles.

Relationship

Complementary: Calcarea.

Compare: Ars. and Verat. in cholera and cholera morbus; Ip. the vegetable analogue.

Verat. follows well in whooping cough and cholera.

Apis and Zinc. in convulsions from suppressed exanthems.

Aggravation

Cold air; cold wind; at night; suppressed foot-sweat or exanthem.

Amelioration

Nausea, vomiting and cough, by a swallow of cold water.

CYCLAMEN EUROPAEUM

Sow Bread   *Primulaceae*

Best suited for leuco-phlegmatic persons with anemic or chlorotic conditions; easily fatigued, and in consequence not inclined to any kind of labor; feeble or suspended functions of organs or special senses.

Pale, chlorotic; deranged menses (Ferr., Puls.); accompanied by vertigo, headache, dim vision.

Pains; pressive, drawing or tearing of parts where bones lie near the surface.

CYCLAMEN EUROPAEUM

Ailments: From suppressed grief and terrors of conscience; from duty not done or bad act committed.

Great sadness and peevishness, irritable, morose, ill-humored; inclined to weep; desire for solitude; *aversion to open air* (reverse of Puls.).

Headache in anemic patients, with flickering before eyes or dim vision, on rising in morning.

Flickering before eyes, fiery sparks, as of various colors, glittering needles, dim vision of fog or smoke.

Satiety after a few mouthfuls (Lyc.), food then becomes repugnant, causes nausea in throat and palate.

Saliva and all food has a salty taste; pork disagrees.

Menses: Too early; too profuse, black and clotted; membranous (too late, pale, scanty, Puls.); better during flow (worse, Cimic., Puls.).

Burning sore pain in heels, when sitting standing or walking in open air (Agar., Caust., Valer., Phyt.).

Relationship

Compare: Puls., Chin., Ferr., in chlorosis, and anemic affections; Croc., Thuja as if something alive in abdomen.

Aggravation

Open air; cold water; cold bathing; menses < sitting and lying at night.

Amelioration

In a warm room; in-doors; menses > walking (leucorrhea, < sitting, > walking, Cact., Cocc.).

DIGITALIS PURPUREA

Foxglove   *Scrophulariaceae*

Sudden flushes of heat, followed by great nervous weakness and irregular intermitting pulse, occurring at the climacteric; < by least motion.

Weak heart without valvular complications.

Sensation as if heart would stop beating if she moved (Cocaine.; fears that unless constantly on the move heart will cease beating, Gels.).

Faintness or sinking at the stomach; exhaustion; extreme prostration; feels as if he were dying.

Nightly emissions, with great weakness of genitals after coitus.

Great weakness of chest, cannot bear to talk (Stann.).

Stools; very light, ash-colored; delayed, chalky (Chel., Podo.); almost white (Calc., Chin.); pipe-stem stool; involuntary.

Pulse full, irregular, **very slow and weak; intermitting every third, fifth or seventh beat.**

Face pale, death-like appearance and bluish-red.

Blueness of skin, eyelids, lips, tongue; cyanosis.

Distended veins on lids, ears, lips and tongue.

Respiration irregular, difficult, deep sighing.

The fingers "go to sleep" frequently and easily.

Dropsy: Post-scarlatinal; in Bright's disease; with suppression of urine; of internal and external parts; with fainting when there are organic affections of the heart (with soreness in uterine region, Conv.).

Fatal syncope may occur when being raised to upright position.

Relationship

Cinchona antidotes the direct action of Digitalis and increases the anxiety.

Aggravation

When sitting, especially when sitting erect; motion.

DIOSCOREA VILLOSA

Wild Yam   *Dioscoreaceae*

Persons of feeble digestive powers, old or young.

Flatulence after meals or after eating, especially of tea drinkers; are often subject to violent colic.

Griping pains in abdomen about umbilicus.

Violent twisting colic, occurring in regular paroxysms, as if intestines were grasped and twisted by a powerful hand.

Colic pains < *from bending forward and while lying;* > on standing erect or bending backwards (rev. of Coloc.).

Emissions during sleep; vivid dreams of women all night (Staph.); knees weak; genitals cold, great despondency (Staph.).

Felons; early when pains are sharp and agonizing, when pricking is first felt; nails brittle.

Disposition to paronychia (Hep).

Relationship

Compare: Coloc., Phos., Podo., Rhus-t., Sil.

Aggravation

Lying; sitting; *bending double*.

Amelioration

Motion; walking difficult; compelled to walk even though tired.

DIPHTHERINUM

Homoeopathic Antitoxin　　　　　　　　*A Nosode*

Especially adapted to the strumous diathesis; scrofulous, psoric or tuberculous persons, prone to catarrhal affections of throat and respiratory mucous membranes.

Patients with weak or exhausted vitality hence are extremely susceptible to the diphtheritic virus; when the attack from the onset tends to malignancy (Lac-c., Merc-cy.).

Painless diphtheria; symptoms almost or entirely objective; patient too weak, apathetic or too prostrated to complain; sopor or stupor, but easily aroused when spoken to (Bapt., Sulph.).

DIPHTHERINUM

Dark red swelling of tonsils and palatine arches; parotid and cervical glands greatly swollen; breath and discharges from throat, nose and mouth very offensive; tongue swollen, very red, little coating.

Diphtheritic membrane, thick, dark gray or brownish-black; temperature low or subnormal, pulse weak and rapid; extremities cold and marked debility; patient lies in a semi-stupid condition; eyes dull, besotted (Apis, Bapt.).

Epistaxis or profound prostration from every onset of attack (Ail., Apis, Carb-ac.); collapse almost at the very beginning (Crot-t., Merc-cy.); pulse weak, rapid and vital reaction very low.

Swallows without pain, but fluids are vomited or returned by the nose; breath horribly offensive.

Laryngeal diphtheria, after Chlor., Kali-bi., or Lac-c. fail; post-diphtheritic paralysis, after Caust., Gels., fail.

When the patient from the first seems doomed, and *the most carefully selected remedies fail to relieve or permanently improve.*

The above are cured symptoms, verifications which the author has found guiding and reliable for twenty-five years.

The remedy is prepared, like all nosodes and animal poisons, according to the Homoeopathic Pharmacopoeia, and like all homoeopathic remedies is entirely safe when given to the sick.

Like all the nosodes it is practically worthless in potencies below the 30th; its curative value also increases with increase of potency from the 200th to the M and C.M. **It need not and should not be repeated too frequently.** It will cure in every case that the crude antitoxin will and is not only easy to administer, but safe and entirely free from dangerous sequelle. Besides, it is homoeopathic.

The author has used it for twenty-five years as a prophylactic and has never known a second case of diphtheria to occur in a family after it had been administered. The profession is asked to put it to the test and publish the failures to the world.

DROSERA ROTUNDIFOLIA

Sundew   *Droseraceae*

Whooping cough with violent paroxysms which follow each other rapidly, is scarcely able to get breath (wakes at 6-7 a.m. and does not cease coughing until a large quantity of tenacious mucus is raised, Coc-c.; profuse epistaxis during every paroxysm, Ind.; "minute gun" during the day whooping at night, Cor-r.).

Deep sounding, hoarse barking cough (Verb.), < after midnight, during or after measles; spasmodic, with gagging, retching and vomiting (Bry., Kali-c.).

Constant, titillating cough in children, begins as soon as head touches pillow at night (Bell., Hyos., Rumx.).

Nocturnal cough of young persons in phthisis; bloody or purulent sputa.

Cough: < by warmth, drinking, singing, laughing, weeping, **lying down,** *after midnight.*

During cough; vomiting of water; mucus, and often bleeding from the nose and mouth (Cupr.).

Sensation of feather in larynx, exciting cough.

Diseases prevailing during epidemic pertussis.

Clergyman's sore throat; with rough, scraping, dry sensation deep in the fauces; voice horse, deep, toneless, cracked, requires exertion to speak (Arum-t.).

Constriction and crawling in larynx; hoarseness, and yellow or green sputa.

Laryngeal phthisis following whooping cough (bronchial catarrh following, Coc-c.).

Relationship

Complementary: To Nux vomica.

Follows well: After Samb., Sulph., Verat.

Is followed: By, Calc., Puls., Sulph.

Compare: Cina, Cor-r., Cupr., Ip., Samb. in spasmodic coughs. Often relieves the constant distressing night cough in tuberculosis.

Hahnemann says (Mat. Med. Pura) "One single dose of 30th potency is sufficient to cure entirely epidemic whooping cough. The cure takes place surely between seven and eight days. Never give a second dose immediately after the first; it would not only prevent the good effect of the former, but would be injurious."

DULCAMARA

Bitter-sweet *Solanaceae*

Adapted to persons of phlegmatic scrofulous constitutions; restless, irritable.

Catarrhal rheumatism or skin affections, brought on or aggravated by exposure to cold, damp, rainy weather, or sudden changes in hot weather (Bry.).

Increased secretion of mucous membranes; perspiration being suppressed from cold.

Patients living or working in a damp, cold basement, or a milk dairy (Aran., Ars., Nat-s.).

Mental confusion; cannot find the right word for anything.

Skin is delicate, sensitive to cold, liable to eruptions, especially urticaria; every time patient takes cold or is long exposed to cold.

Anasarca; after ague, rheumatism, scarlet fever.

Dropsy: After suppressed sweat; suppressed eruptions; exposure to cold.

Diarrhea: From taking cold in damp places, or during damp, foggy weather; change from warm to cold weather (Bry.).

Catarrhal ischuria in grown-up children, with milky urine; *from wading with bare feet in cold water; involuntary.*

Rash before the menses (Con.; during profuse menses, Bell., Graph.).

DULCAMARA

Urticaria over whole body, no fever; itching burns after scratching; < in warmth, > in cold.

Thick brown-yellow crusts on scalp, face, forehead, temples, chin; with reddish borders, bleeding when scratched.

Warts, fleshy, large, smooth; on face or back of hands and fingers (Thuj.).

Relationship

Complementary: To, Baryta carb., Kali-s.

Incompatible: With Acet-ac., Bell., Lach.

Should not be used before or after.

Follows well: After, Calc., Bry., Lyc., Rhus-t., Sep.

Similar: To Merc. in ptyalism, glandular swellings, bronchitis, diarrhea; susceptibility to weather changes; night pains; to Kali-s. the chemical analogue.

For the bad effects or abuse of mercury.

Aggravation

From cold in general; cold air; cold wet weather; suppressed menstruation, eruptions, sweat.

Amelioration

From moving about (Ferr., Rhus-t.).

EQUISETUM HYEMALE

Scouring Rush *Equisetaceae*

Severe dull pain in the bladder, as from distention, not > after urinating.

Frequent and intolerable urging to urinate, with severe pain *at close of urination* (Berb., Sars., Thuj.).

Constant desire to urinate; large quantity of clear, watery urine, without > (scanty, a few drops, Apis, Canth.).

Sharp, burning, cutting pain in urethra while urinating.

Paralysis of bladder in old women.

Enuresis diurna et nocturna; profuse watery urine, where habit is the only ascertainable cause.

Relationship
Compare: Apis, Canth., Ferr-p., Puls., Squill.

EUPATORIUM PERFOLIATUM

Boneset *Compositae*

Adapted to diseases of old people; *worn-out* constitutions, *especially from inebriety;* cachexia, from prolonged or frequent attacks of bilious or intermittent fevers.

EUPATORIUM PERFOLIATUM

Bruised feeling, as if broken, all over the body (Arn., Bell-p., Pyrog.).

Bone pains affecting back, head, chest, limbs, especially the wrists, as if dislocated. The more general and severe, the better adapted (compare, Bry., Merc.).

Painful soreness of eyeballs; coryza, aching in every bone; great prostration in epidemic influenza (Lac-c.).

Pains come quickly and go away as quickly (Bell., Mag-p., Eup-pur.).

Vertigo; sensation as if falling to the left (cannot turn the head to the left for fear of falling, Coloc.).

Cough: Chronic; loose with hectic; chest sore, must support it with hands (Bry., Nat-c.); < at night; following measles or suppressed intermittents.

Fever: Chill at 9 a.m. one day, at noon the next day; bitter vomiting at close of chill; drinking hastens chill and causes vomiting ; **bone pains,** *before and during chill.*

Insatiable thirst before and during chill and fever; knows chill is coming *because he cannot drink enough.*

Relationship

Is followed well: By, Nat-m. and Sep.

Compare: Chel., Podo., Lyc., in jaundiced conditions.

Bryonia is the nearest analogue, having free sweat, but pains keep patient quiet; while Eup-per. has scanty sweat and pains make patient restless.

EUPHRASIA

Eyebright   *Scrophularaceae*

Bad effects from falls, contusions or mechanical injuries of external parts (Arn.).

Catarrhal affections of mucous membranes, especially of the eyes and nose.

Profuse **acrid lachrymation,** with profuse, **bland coryza** (reverse of All-c.).

The eyes water all the time and are agglutinated in the morning; margins of lids red, swollen, burning.

Profuse fluent coryza in morning with violent cough and abundant expectoration, < from exposure to warm south wind.

When attempting to clear the throat of an offensive mucus in the morning, gagging until he vomits the breakfast just eaten (Bry.).

Profuse expectoration of mucus by voluntary hawking, < on rising in morning.

Amenorrhea, with catarrhal symptoms of eyes and nose; profuse acrid lachrymation.

Menses: Painful, regular, **now lasting only one hour;** or late, scanty, short, lasting only one day (Bar-c.).

Pertussis: *Excessive lachrymation during cough; cough only in day time* (Ferr., Nat-m.).

Relationship

Similar: To, Puls. in affections of the eyes; reverse of All-c. in lachrymation and coryza.

Aggravation

In the evening, in bed, indoors, warmth, moisture; *after exposure to south wind;* when touched (Hep.).

FERRUM METALLICUM

Iron *The Element*

Persons of sanguine temperament; pettish, quarrelsome, disputative, easily excited, least contradiction angers (Anac., Cocc., Ign.); > from mental exertion.

Irritability; slight noises like crackling of paper drive him to despair (Asar., Tarent.).

Women who are weak, delicate, chlorotic, yet have a fiery red face.

Extreme paleness of the face, lips and mucous membranes *which become red and flushed on the least pain, emotion or exertion.* Blushing (Aml-ns., Coca).

Erethitic chlorosis, worse in winter.

Red parts become white; face, lips, tongue and mucous membrane of mouth.

Vertigo: With balancing sensation, as if on water; *on seeing flowing water;* when walking over water, as when crossing a bridge (Lyss.); on descending (Borx., Sanic.).

Headache: Hammering, beating, pulsating pains, must lie down; with aversion to eating or drinking. For two, three or four days every two or three weeks.

FERRUM METALLICUM

Menses: Too early, too profuse, too long lasting, with fiery red face; ringing in the ears; intermit two or three days and then return; *flow pale, watery, debilitating.*

Hemorrhagic diathesis; blood bright red, coagulates easily (Ferr-p., Ip., Phos.).

Regurgitation and eructation of food in mouthfuls (Alum.), without nausea.

Canine hunger, or loss of appetite, with extreme dislike for all food.

Vomiting: *Immediately after midnight;* of ingesta, as soon as food is eaten; leaves table suddenly and with one effort vomits everything eaten, can sit down and eat again; sour, acid (Lyc., Sul-ac.).

Diarrhea: Undigested stools at night, or **while eating or drinking** (Crot-t.); painless with a good appetite; of consumptives.

Constipation: From intestinal atony; ineffectual urging; stools hard, difficult, followed by backache or cramping pain in rectum; prolapsus recti of children; itching of anus at night.

Always feels better *by walking slowly about,* although weakness obliges the patient to lie down.

Cough only in the day time (Euphr.); relieved by lying down; > by eating (Spong.).

Dropsy: After loss of vital fluids; abuse of quinine; suppressed intermittent (Carb-v., Chin.).

Relationship

Complementary: To, Alum., Chin.

Chin: The vegetable analogue follows well in nearly all diseases, acute or chronic.

Should never be given in syphilis; always aggravates the condition.

Aggravation
At night; at rest, especially while sitting still.

Amelioration
Walking slowly about; in summer.

FLUORICUM ACIDUM

Hydrofluoric Acid   *HF*

Complaints of old age, or of premature old age; in syphilitic mercurial dyscrasia; *young people look old.*

Increased ability to exercise without danger (Coca); is less affected by excessive heat of summer or cold of winter.

Old cicatrices become red around edges, and threaten to become open ulcers (Caust., Graph.).

Varicose veins and ulcers, obstinate, long standing cases, in women who have borne many children.

Caries and necrosis, especially of long bones, psoric or syphilitic, abuse of mercury or silica (Agn.).

Nevus flat, of children (right temple); capillary aneurysm (compare, Calc-f., Tub.).

Ulcers: Red edges and vesicles; decubitus; copious discharge; < from warmth, > from cold; violent pains, like streaks of lightning, confined to a small spot.

Rapid caries of teeth; fistula dentalis or lachrymalis; exostosis of bones of face (Hecla).

Relationship

Complementary: Coca, Sil.

Follows well: After, Ars. in ascites of drunkards; after, Kali-c, in hip disease; after, Coff., Staph. in sensitive teeth; after, Ph-ac., in diabetes; after, Sil., Symph. in bone diseases; after, Spong. in goitre.

GELSEMIUM

Yellow Jasmine *Loganiaceae*

For children, young people, especially women of a nervous hysterical temperament (Croc., Ign.).

Complete relaxation and prostration of the whole muscular system, with motor paralysis.

Excitable, irritable, sensitive; for the nervous affections of onanists of both sexes (Kali-p.).

Bad effects from fright, fear, exciting news and sudden emotions (Ign.; from pleasant surprise, Coff.).

Fear of death (Ars.); utter lack of courage.

The anticipation of any unusual ordeal preparing for church, theatre, or to meet an engagement, brings

GELSEMIUM

on diarrhea; stage fright, nervous dread of appearing in public (Arg-n.).

General depression *from heat of sun or summer.*

Weakness and trembling; of tongue, hands, legs; of the entire body.

Desire to be quiet, to be let alone; does not wish to speak or have any one near her, even in the person be silent (Ign.).

Vertigo, *spreading from the occiput* (Sil.); with diplopia, dim vision, loss of sight; seems intoxicated when trying to move.

Children: Fear of falling, grasp the crib or seize the nurse (Borx., Sanic.).

Headache: Preceded by blindness (Kali-bi.), > by profuse urination.

Lack of muscular co-ordination; *confused;* muscles refuse to obey the will.

Headache: *Beginning in the cervical spine;* pains extend over the head, causing a bursting sensation in forehead and eye balls (Sang., Sil., begins in same way, but semi-lateral); < by mental exertion; from smoking; heat of sun; lying with head low.

Sensation of band around the head above eyes (Carb-ac., Sulph.); scalp sore to touch.

Fears that unless on the move heart will cease beating (fears it would cease beating if she moved, Dig.).

Slow pulse of old age.

Great heaviness of the eyelids; cannot keep them open (Caust., Graph., Sep.).

Chill without thirst, especially along the spine, *running up and down the back* in rapid, wave-like succession from sacrum to occiput.

Relationship

Compare: Bapt. in threatening typhoid fever; Ip. in dumb ague, after suppression by quinine.

Aggravation

Damp weather; before a thunderstorm; mental emotion or excitement *bad news; tobacco smoking;* when *thinking of his ailments;* when spoken to of his loss.

GLONOINUM

Nitro-glycerine $C_3H_5(NO_2)O_3$

Nervous temperament: Plethoric, florid, sensitive women; persons readily affected.

Bad effects of mental excitement, fright, fear, mechanical injuries and their later consequences; from having the hair cut (Acon., Bell.).

Head troubles: From working under gas-light, when heat falls on head; cannot bear heat about the head, heat of stove or *walking in the sun* (Lach., Nat-c.).

Cerebral congestion, or alternate congestion of the head and heart.

Head: Feels enormously large; as if skull were too small for brain; **sunstroke and sun headache;** increases and decreases everyday with the sun (Kalm., Nat-c.).

GLONOINUM

Terrific shock in the head, synchronous with the pulse. Throbbing, pulsating headache; holds head with both hands; could not lie down, "the pillow would beat".

Brain feels *too large, full, bursting;* blood seems to be pumped upwards; *throbs at every jar, step, pulse.*

Intense congestion of brain from delayed or suppressed menses; **headache in place of menses.**

Headache: Occurring after profuse uterine hemorrhage: *rush of blood to head,* in pregnant women.

Violent palpitation, with throbbing in carotids; heart's action labored, oppressed; blood seems to rush to heart, and rapidly to head.

Convulsions of children from cerebral congestion; meningitis, during dentition, cases that seem to call for Belladonna.

Children get sick in the evening when sitting before an open coal fire, or falling asleep there.

Flushes of heat; at the climacteric (Aml-ns., Bell., Lach.); with the catamenia (Ferr., Sang.).

Relationship

Compare: Aml-ns., Bell., Ferr., Gels., Meli., Stram.

Aggravation

In the sun, exposure to sun's rays; gas-light; overheating; jar; stooping; ascending; touch of hat; having the hair cut.

GRAPHITES

Black Lead   **Amorphous Carbon**

Suited to women, inclined to obesity, who suffer from habitual constipation; with a history of delayed menstruation.

"What Pulsatilla is at puberty, Graphites is at the climacteric."

Excessive cautiousness; timid, hesitates; unable to decide about anything (Puls.).

Fidgety while sitting at work (Zinc.).

Sad, despondent; *music makes her weep;* thinks of nothing but death (music is intolerable, Nat-c., Sab.).

Eczema of lids; eruption moist and fissured; lids red and margins covered with scales or crusts.

Sexual debility from sexual abuse.

Menses: Too scanty, pale, late with violent colic; irregular; delayed from getting feet wet (Puls.).

Morning sickness during menstruation; very weak and prostrated (Alumn., Carb-an., Cocc.).

Leucorrhea: Acrid, excoriating; occurs **in gushes day and night;** before and after menses (before Sep.; after Kreos.).

Hard cicatrices remaining after mammary abscess, retarding the flow of milk; cancer of breast, from old scars and repeated abscesses.

Unhealthy skin; *every injury suppurates* (Hep.); old cicatrices break open again; *eruptions upon the ears,* between fingers and toes and on various parts of body, from which oozes **a watery, transparent, sticky fluid.**

The nails are brittle, crumbling, deformed (Ant-c.); painful, sore, as if ulcerated; thick and crippled.

Cracks or fissures, in ends of fingers, nipples, labial commissures; of anus; between the toes.

Burning round spot on vertex (Calc., Sulph.; cold spot, Sep., Verat.).

Cataleptic condition; conscious, but without power to move or speak.

Takes cold easily, sensitive to draft of air (Borx., Calc., Hep., Nux-v.). Suffering parts emaciate.

Hears better when in a noise; when riding in a carriage or car, when there is a rumbling sound (Nit-ac.).

Diarrhea: Stools brown, fluid, mixed with undigested substances, and of an intolerable odor often caused by suppressed eruptions (Psor.).

Chronic constipation; stool difficult, large, hard, knotty, with lumps united by mucus threads; *too large* (Sulph.); smarting sore pain in anus after stool.

Children: Impudent, teasing, laugh at reprimands.

Sensation of cobwebs on forehead, tries hard to brush it off (Bar-c., Borx., Brom., Ran-s.).

Phlegmonous erysipelas: Of face, with burning, stinging pain; commencing on right side, going to left; after application of iodine.

Decided aversion to coition (both sexes).

Relationship

Complementary: Caust., Hep., Lyc.

Graphites follows well: After Lyc., Puls.; after Calc. in obesity of young women with large amount of unhealthy adipose tissue; follows Sulph. well in skin affections; after Sepia in gushing leucorrhea.

Similar: To Lyc., Puls., in menstrual troubles.

Aggravation

At night, during and after menstruation.

HAMAMELIS VIRGINICA

Witch Hazel *Hamamelaceae*

The shrub flowers from September to November, when the leaves are falling. The seeds mature the following summer.

It is adapted to venous hemorrhage from every orifice of the body; nose, lungs, bowels, uterus, bladder.

Venous congestion: Passive, of skin and mucous membranes; phlebitis, varicose veins; ulcers, varicose, with stinging, pricking pain; hemorrhoids.

Patients, subject to varicose veins, taking cold easily from every exposure, especially in warm, moist air.

"Is the Aconite of the venous capillary system."

Bruised soreness of affected parts (Arn.); rheumatism, articular and muscular.

HAMAMELIS VIRGINICA

Wounds: Incised, lacerated, contused; injuries from falls; checks hemorrhage, removes pain and soreness (Arn.).

Chronic effects of mechanical injuries (Con.).

Traumatic conjunctivitis; suggillations, or extravasations into chambers of eye; from severe coughing; *intense soreness* (Arn., Calen., Led.).

Nosebleed: Flow passive, long-lasting, blood non-coagulable (Crot-t.); profuse > headache (Mel.); idiopathic, traumatic, vicarious, of childhood.

Hemorrhage: Profuse, dark, grumous, from ulceration of bowels (Crot-h.); uterine, active or passive; after a fall or rough riding; vicarious menstruation; no mental anxiety.

Hemoptysis: Tickling cough, with taste of blood or sulphur; venous, without effort or coughing; sometimes monthly, for years.

Profuse discharges, which simulate a hemorrhage, and form a drain upon system as severe as loss of blood.

Hemorrhoids: Bleeding profusely; with burning; soreness, fullness, heaviness; as if back would break; urging to stool; bluish color; anus feels sore and raw.

Menses: Flow, dark and profuse; with soreness in abdomen; after a blow on ovary, or a fall; all suffering < at menstrual period (Cimic., Puls.).

Uterine hemorrhage active or passive; from jolting while riding over rough roads; bearing down pain in back.

After hemorrhage from piles, prostration out of all proportion to amount of blood lost (Hydr.).

Bad effects from loss of blood (Chin).

Relationship

Complementary: Ferrum, in hemorrhages and the hemorrhagic diathesis.

Compare: Arn., Calen., for traumatic, and to hasten absorption of intraocular hemorrhage.

HELLEBORUS NIGER

Christmas Rose   *Ranunculaceae*

Weakly, delicate, psoric children; prone to brain troubles (Bell., Calc., Tub.); with serous effusion.

Melancholy; woeful; despairing; silent with anguish; after typhoid; in girls at puberty, or when menses fail to return after appearing.

Irritable, easily angered; consolation < (Ign., Nat-m., Sep., Sil.); does not want to be disturbed (Gels., Nat-m.).

Unconscious; stupid; answers slowly when questioned; a picture of acute idiocy (of chronic, Bar-c.).

Brain symptoms during dentition (Bell., Podo.); threatening effusion (Apis, Tub.).

Meningitis: Acute, cerebro-spinal, tubercular, with exudation; paralysis more or less complete; with the cri encephalique.

Vacant, thoughtless starting; *eye wide open;* insensible to light; pupils dilated, or alternately contracted and dilated.

Soporous sleep, with screams, shrieks, starts.

Hydrocephalus, post-scarlatinal or tubercular which develops rapidly (Apis, Sulph., Tub.); automatic motion of one arm and leg.

Convulsions with extreme coldness of body, except head or occiput which may be hot (Arn.).

Greedily swallows cold water; bites spoon, but remains unconscious.

Chewing motion of the mouth; corners of mouth sore, cracked; nostrils dirty and sooty, dry.

Constantly pricking his lips, clothes, or boring into his nose with his finger (while perfectly conscious, Arum-t.).

Boring head into pillow; rolling from side to side; beating head with hands.

Diarrhea: During acute hydrocephalus, dentition, pregnancy; watery, clear, tenacious, colorless mucus; white, jelly-like mucus; like frog spawn; involuntary.

Urine: **Red, black, scanty, coffee-ground sediment; suppressed** in brain troubles and dropsy; albuminous.

Dropsy: Of brain, chest, abdomen; after scarlatina, intermittents; with fever, debility, *suppressed urine;* from suppressed exanthemata (Apis, Zinc.).

Relationship

Compare: Apis, Apoc., Ars., Bell., Bry., Dig., Lach., Sulph., Tub., Zinc. in brain or meningeal affections.

HELONIAS DIOICA

Unicorn Plant   *Melanthaceae*

For women: With *prolapsus from atony*, enervated by indolence and luxury; *worn out with hard work, mental or physical;* overtaxed muscles burn and ache; so tired cannot sleep.

Always better when occupied, when not thinking of the ailment (Calc-p., Ox-ac.).

Restless, must be continually moving about.

Irritable, fault finding; cannot endure least contradiction or receive least suggestion (Anac.).

Profound melancholy; deep, mental depression.

Diabetes: First stages; urine profuse, clear, saccharine; lips dry, stick together; great thirst; restlessness; emaciation; irritable and melancholy.

Albuminuria: Acute or chronic; during pregnancy; with great weakness, languor, drowsiness; unusually tired, yet knows no reason.

Menses: Too early, too profuse, from uterine atony in women enfeebled by loss of blood; when patients lose more blood than is made in intermenstrual period; breasts swollen, nipples painful and tender (Con., Lac-c.). Flow passive, dark, clotted, offensive.

Sensation of soreness and heaviness in pelvis (Lappa); *a consciousness of the womb,* feels it move when she moves, *it is so sore and tender* (Lyss.).

For the bad effects of abortions and miscarriages.

Relationship

Compare: Alet., Ferr., Lil-t., Ph-ac.

Similar: To, Alet. in debility from prolapsus, protracted illness, defective nutrition.

HEPAR SULPHURIS

Sulphuret of Lime   *Ca.S*

For torpid lymphatic constitutions; persons with light hair and complexion, slow to act, muscles soft and flabby.

The slightest injury causes suppuration (Graph., Merc.).

Diseases where the system has been injured by the abuse of mercury.

In diseases where suppuration seems inevitable, Hepar may open the abscess and hasten the cure

Oversensitive, physically and mentally; the slightest cause irritates him; quick, hasty speech and hasty drinking.

Patient is peevish, angry at the least trifle; hypochondriacal; unreasonably anxious.

Extremely sensitive to cold air, imagines he can feel the air if a door is opened in the next room; must be wrapped up to the face even in hot weather (Psor.); cannot bear to be uncovered (Nux-v.; cannot bear to be covered, Camph., Sec.); takes cold from slightest exposure to fresh air (Tub.).

Urine: Flow impeded, *voided slowly, without force, drops vertically;* is obliged to wait awhile before it passes; bladder weak, is unable to finish, seems as if some urine always remains (Alum., Sil.).

Cough: *When any part of the body is uncovered* (Rhus-t.); **croupy, choking, strangling;** *from exposure to dry west wind,* the land wind (Acon.).

Asthma: Breathing, anxious, wheezing, rattling; short, deep breathing, threatens suffocation; must bend head back and sit up; after suppressed eruption (Psor.).

Croup: After exposure *to dry cold wind* (Acon.); deep, rough, barking cough, with hoarseness and rattling of mucus; < cold air, cold drinks, before midnight or towards morning.

Sensation of a splinter, fish bone or plug in the throat (Arg-n., Nit-ac.); quinsy, when suppuration threatens; chronic hypertrophy, with hardness of hearing (Bar-c., Lyc., Plb., Psor.).

The skin is **very sensitive to touch,** cannot bear even clothes to touch affected parts (Lach.; sensitive to slightest touch, but can bear hard pressure, Chin.).

Skin affections **extremely sensitive to touch,** the pain often causing fainting.

Ulcers, herpes, surrounded by little pimples or pustules and spread by coalescing.

Middle of lower lip cracked (Am-c., Nat-m.; cracks in commissures, Cund.).

HEPAR SULPHURIS 151

Eyeballs: Sore to touch; pain as if they would be pulled back into head (Olnd., Par.).

Diarrhea: Of children with sour smell (Calc., Mag-c.; child and stool have a sour smell, Rheum); clay-colored stool (Calc., Podo.).

Sweats: Profusely day and night without relief; perspiration sour; offensive; easily, on every mental or physical exertion (Psor., Sep.).

Relationship

Complementary: To, Calendula in injuries of soft parts.

Hepar antidotes: Bad effects of mercury and other metals; iodine, iodide of potash, cod-liver oil; renders patients less susceptible to atmospheric changes and cold air.

Compare: The psoric skin affections of Sulphur are dry, itching, > by scratching, and not sensitive to touch; while in Hepar the skin is unhealthy, suppurating, moist, and extremely sensitive to touch.

Aggravation

Lying on painful side (Kali-c., Iod.); cold air; uncovering; eating or drinking cold things; touching affected parts; abuse of mercury.

Amelioration

Warmth in general (Ars.); wrapping up warmly, especially the head (Psor., Sil.); *in damp, wet weather* (Caust., Nux-v.; reverse of, Nat-s.).

HYDRASTIS CANADENSIS

Golden Seal   *Ranunculaceae*

For debilitated persons, with viscid mucus discharges.

Cachectic or malignant dyscrasia, with marked derangement of gastric and hepatic functions; broken down by excessive use of alcohol.

Cancer breast; hard, adherent; skin mottled, puckered; pains knife-like, sharp, cutting; nipple retracted.

Nursing sore mouth; tongue large, shows imprint of teeth.

Leucorrhea: Ropy, thick, viscid, yellow; hanging from os in long strings (Kali-bi.); pruritus.

Profuse discharge of thick, yellow, stringy mucus from nasal passages (Cor-r.).

Hawks yellow, viscid mucus from posterior nares and fauces; ulceration after mercury or chlorate of potash; syphilitic angina.

HYOSCYAMUS NIGER

Henbane   *Solanaceae*

Persons of sanguine temperament; who are irritable, nervous, hysterical.

HYOSCYAMUS NIGER

Convulsions: Of children, from fright or the irritation of intestinal worms (Cina); during labor; during the puerperal stage; after meals, child vomits, sudden shriek, then insensible.

Diseases with increased cerebral activity, but *non-inflammatory in type;* hysteria or delirium tremens; delirium, with restlessness, jumps out of bed, tries to escape; makes irrelevant answers; thinks he is in the wrong place; talks of imaginary doings, but has no wants and makes no complaints.

In delirium, Hyoscyamus occupies a place midway between Belladonna and Stramonium; lacks the constant cerebral congestion of the former and the fierce rage and maniacal delirium of the latter.

Spasms: Without consciousness, very restless; *every muscle in the body twitches, from the eyes to the toes* (with consciousness, Nux-v.).

Fears: Being alone; poison; being bitten; being sold; to eat or drink; to take what is offered; *suspicious,* of some plot.

Bad effects of unfortunate love; with jealousy, rage, incoherent speech or inclination to laugh at everything; often followed by epilepsy.

Lascivious mania: *immodesty, will not be covered,* kicks off the clothes, *exposes the person;* sings obscene songs; lies naked in bed and chatters.

Cough: Dry, nocturnal, spasmodic; < *when lying down, relieved by sitting up* (Dros.); < at night, after eating, drinking, talking, singing (Dros., Phos.; > when lying down, Mang-met.).

Intense sleeplessness of irritable, excitable persons from business embarrassments, often imaginary.

Paralysis of bladder; after labor, with retention or incontinence of urine; no desire to urinate in lying - in women (Arn., Op.).

Fever: Pneumonia, scarlatina, *rapidly becomes typhoid;* sensorium clouded, staring eyes, grasping at flocks or picking bed clothes, teeth covered with sordes, tongue dry and unwieldy; involuntary stool and urine; subsultus tendinum.

Relationship

Compare: Bell., Stram. and Verat.

Phos. often cures lasciviousness when Hyos. fails.

Nux-v. or Opium in hemoptysis of drunkards.

Follows: Bell. well in deafness after apoplexy.

Aggravation

At night; during menses; mental affections; jealousy, unhappy love; when lying down.

HYPERICUM PERFORATUM

St. John's Wort *Hypericaceae*

Mechanical injuries of spinal cord; bad effects of spinal concussion; pains, after a fall on coccyx.

Punctured, incised or lacerated wounds; sore, painful (Led.; contused wounds, Arn., Ham.), especially if of long duration.

Injuries from treading on nails, needles, pins, splinters (Led.); from rat-bites; *prevents lockjaw.*

Preserves integrity of torn and lacerated members when almost entirely separated from body (Calen.).

Injury to **parts rich in sentient nerves** – fingers, toes, matrices of nails, palms or soles—where the intolerable pain shows nerves are severely involved; of tissues of animal life, as hands and feet.

Nervous depression following wounds or surgical operations; removes bad effect of shock, of fright, of mesmerism.

Always modifies and sometimes arrests ulceration and sloughing (Calen.). Crushed, mashed fingertips. Tetanus after traumatic injuries (compare, Phys.).

Vertigo: Sensation as if head became suddenly elongated; at night, with urging to urinate.

Headache: After a fall upon the occiput, with sensation *as if being lifted up high into the air;* great anxiety lest she fall from this height.

Spine: After a fall; slightest motion of arms or neck extorts cries; spine very sensitive to touch.

Bunions and corns when pain is excruciating, showing nerve involvement.

Convulsions; after blows on head or concussion.

Relationship

Compare: Arn., Calen., Ruta, Staph.

In wounds where formerly Acon. and Arn. were given alternately, Hypericum cures.

IGNATIA

St. Ignatius Bean   *Loganiaceae*

Especially suited to nervous temperament; women of a sensitive, easily excited nature; dark hair and skin but mild disposition, quick to perceive, rapid in execution. In striking contrast with the fair complexion, yielding, lachrymose, but slow and indecisive, Pulsatilla).

The remedy of great contradictions: The roaring in ears > by music; the piles > when walking; sore throat feels > when swallowing; empty feeling in stomach not > by eating; cough < the more he coughs; cough on standing still during a walk (Astac.); spasmodic laughter from grief; sexual desire with impotency; *thirst during a chill,* no thirst in the fever; the color changes in the face when at rest.

Mental conditions rapidly, in an almost incredibly short time, change from joy to sorrow, from laughing to weeping (Coff., Croc., Nux-m.); **moody.**

Persons mentally and physically exhausted by **long-concentrated grief.**

Involuntary sighing (Lach.); with a weak, empty feeling at pit of stomach; not > by eating (Hydr., Sep.),

Bad effects of anger, grief, or disappointed love (Calc-p., Hyos.); broods in solitude over imaginary trouble.

Desire to be alone.

Finely sensitive mood, delicate consciousness.

IGNATIA

Inconstant, impatient, irresolute, quarrelsome.

Amiable in disposition if feeling well, but easily disturbed by very slight emotion; *easily offended.*

The slightest fault finding or contradiction excites anger, and this makes him angry with himself.

Children, when reprimanded, scolded, or sent to bed, get sick or have convulsions in sleep.

Ill-effects, from bad news; from vexation with reserved displeasure; from suppressed mental sufferings; of shame and mortification (Staph.).

Headache, as if a nail was driven out through the side, relieved by lying on it (Coff., Nux-v., Thuj.).

Cannot bear tobacco; smoking, or being in tobacco smoke, produces or aggravates headache.

In talking or chewing, bites inside of cheek.

Sweat on the face on a small spot only while eating.

Oversensitiveness to pain (Coff., Cham.).

Constipation: From carriage riding; of a paralytic origin; with *excessive urging, felt more in upper abdomen* (Verat.); with great pain, dreads to go to closet; in women who are habitual coffee drinkers.

Prolapsus ani from moderate straining at stool, stooping or lifting (Nit-ac., Podo., Ruta); < when the stool is loose.

Hemorrhoids: Prolapse with every stool, have to be replaced; *sharp stitches shoot up the rectum* (Nit-ac.); < for hours after stool (Rat., Sulph.).

Twitching jerkings, even spasms of single limbs or whole body, when falling asleep.

Pain in small, circumscribed spots.

Fever: Red face during chill (Ferr.); chill, *with thirst during chill only;* > by external heat; heat *without thirst,* < by covering (> by covering, Nux-v.).

Complaints return at precisely the same hour.

Ignatia bears the same relation to the diseases of women that Nux-v. does to sanguine, bilious men.

There are many more Ignatia persons in North America than Nux vomica persons. – Hering.

Relationship

Incompatible: Coff., Nux-v., Tab.

The bad effects of Ign. are antidoted by Puls.

Aggravation

From tobacco, coffee, brandy, contact, motion, strong odors, mental emotions, grief.

Amelioration

Warmth, hard pressure (Chin.); swallowing, walking.

IODIUM

Iodine   *The Element*

Persons of scrofulous diathesis, with dark or black hair and eyes; a low cachetic condition, *with profound debility and* **great emaciation** (Abrot.).

IODIUM

Great weakness and loss of breath on going upstairs (Calc.); during the menses (Alum., Carb-an., Cocc.).

Ravenous hunger; eats freely and well, yet loses **flesh all the time** (Abrot., Nat-m., Sanic., Tub.).

Empty eructations from morning to night, as if every particle of food was turned into air (Kali-c.).

Suffers from hunger, must eat every few hours, anxious and worried if he does not eat (Cina, Sulph.); *feels > while eating or after eating,* when stomach is full.

Itching: Low down in the lungs, behind the sternum, causing cough; extends through bronchi to nasal cavity (Coc-c., Con., Phos.).

Hypertrophy and induration of glandular tissue—thyroid, mammae, ovaries, testes, uterus, prostate or other glands—breasts may dwindle and become flabby.

Hard goitre, in dark-haired persons (light-haired, Brom.); feels > after eating.

Palpitation, worse from least exertion (compare Dig.; from least mental exertion, Calc-ar.).

Sensation as if the heart was squeezed together; as if grasped with an iron hand (Cact., Sulph.).

Leucorrhea: Acrid, corrosive, staining and corroding the linen; most abundant at times of menses.

Cancerous degeneration of cervix; cutting pains in abdomen and hemorrhage at every stool.

Constipation, with ineffectual urging > by drinking cold milk.

Croup: Membranous, hoarse, dry cough, worse in

warm, wet weather; with wheezing and sawing respiration (Spong.).

Child grasps the larynx (All-c.); face pale and cold, especially in fleshy children.

Relationship

Complementary: To, Lycopodium.

Compare: Acet-ac., Brom., Con., Kali-bi., Spong. in membranous croup and croupy affections; especially in overgrown boys with scrofulous diathesis.

Follows well: After; Hep., Merc.; is followed by Kali-bi. in croup. Acts best in goitre when given after full moon, or when the moon is waning.—Lippe.

Should not be given during lying-in period, except in high potencies.— Hering.

Aggravation

Warmth; wraping up the head (reverse of, Hep., Psor.).

IPECACUANHA

Ipecac *Rubiaceae*

Adapted to cases where the gastric symptoms predominate (Ant-c., Puls.); *tongue clean* or slightly coated.

In all diseases with constant and continual nausea.

Nausea; *with profuse saliva;* vomiting of white, glairy mucus in large quantities, *without relief;* sleepy

IPECACUANHA

afterwards; worse from stooping; the primary effects of tobacco; of pregnancy.

Stomach: Feels relaxed *as if hanging down* (Ign., Staph.); clutching, squeezing, griping, as from a hand, each finger sharply pressing into intestines; worse from motion.

Flatulent, cutting colic about umbilicus.

Stool: Grassy-green; of white mucus (Colch.); bloody; fermented, foamy, slimy, like frothy molasses.

Autumnal dysentery; cold nights, after hot days (Colch., Merc.).

Asiatic cholera, first symptoms, where nausea and vomiting predominate (Colch.).

Hemorrhage: Active or passive, **bright red** *from all the orifices of the body* (Erig., Mill.); uterine profuse, clotted; heavy, oppressed breathing during; stitches from naval to uterus.

Cutting pains across abdomen from left to right (Lach.; from right to left, Lyc.).

Cough; dry spasmodic, constricted, asthmatic.

Difficulty breathing from least exercise; violent dyspnea with wheezing and anxiety about the stomach.

Whooping cough; *child loses breath,* turns pale, stiff and blue; strangling, with gagging and vomiting of mucus; bleeding from nose or mouth (Indigo).

Cough, with rattling of mucus in bronchi when inspiring (Ant-t.); threatened suffocation from mucus.

Pains as if bones were all torn to pieces (as if broken, Eup-per.).

Intermittent fever: In beginning of irregular cases; **with nausea,** or from gastric disturbance; after abuse of, or suppression from quinine.

Intermittent dyspepsia, every other day at same hour; fever, with persistent nausea.

Oversensitive to heat and cold.

Relationship

Complementary: Cuprum.

Is followed well: By, Ars. in influenza, chills, croup, debility, cholera infantum; by, Ant-t. in foreign bodies in larynx.

Similar: To, Puls., Ant-c., gastric troubles.

Aggravation

Winter and dry weather; warm, moist, south winds (Euphr.); slightest motion.

KALIUM BICHROMICUM

Potassium Bichromate $K_2Cr_2O_7$

Fat, light-haired persons who suffer from catarrhal syphilitic or psoric affections.

Fat, chubby, short-necked children disposed to croup and croupy affections.

Affections of the mucous membranes—eyes, nose, mouth, throat, bronchi; gastro-intestinal and genito-

KALIUM BICHROMICUM

urinary tracts—**discharge of a tough, shringy mucus which adheres to the parts and can be drawn into the long strings** (compare, Hydr., Lyss.).

Complaints occurring in hot weather.

Liability to take cold in open air.

Rheumatism alternating with gastric symptoms, one appearing in the fall and the other in the spring; rheumatism and dysentery alternate (Abrot.).

Pains: *In small spots,* can be covered with point of finger (Ign.); *shift rapidly* from one part to another (Kali-s., Lac-c., Puls.); appear and disappear suddenly (Bell., Ign., Mag-p.).

Neuralgia everyday at same hour (Chinin-s.).

Gastric complaints: Bad effects of beer; loss of appetite; weight in pit of stomach; flatulence; < soon after eating; vomiting of ropy mucus and blood; round ulcer of stomach (Gymno.).

Nose: *Pressive pain in root of nose (in forehead and root of nose,* Stict.); **discharge of plugs, "clinkers";** tough, ropy, green fluid mucus; in clear masses, and has violent pain from occiput to forehead if discharge ceases.

Ulceration of septum, with bloody discharge or large flakes of hard mucus (Alum., Sep., Teucr.).

Diphtheria: Pseudo-membranous deposit, firm, pearly, fibrinous, prone to extend downwards to larynx and trachea (Lac-c.; reverse of, Brom.).

Edematous, bladder-like appearance of uvula; much swelling, but little redness (Rhus-t.).

KALIUM BICHROMICUM

Cough: Violent, rattling, with gagging from viscid mucus in the throat; < when undressing (Hep.).

Croup: *Hoarse, metallic,* with expectoration of tough mucus or fibro-elastic casts in morning on awakening **with dyspnea, > by lying down** (worse when lying down, Aral., Lach.).

Deep-eating ulcers in fauces; often syphilitic.

Headache: *Blurred vision or blindness precedes* the attack (Gels., Lac-d.); must lie down; aversion to light and noise; sight returns as headache increases (Iris, Nat-m., Lac-d.).

Prolapsus uteri, seemingly in hot weather.

Sexual desire absent in fleshy people.

Relationship

Compare: Brom., Hep., Iod. in croupy affections.

After: Canth. or Carb-ac. has removed the scrapings in dysentery.

After: Iod. in croup, when hoarse cough, with tough membrane, general weakness and coldness are present; Calc. in acute or chronic nasal catarrh.

Ant-t. follows well in catarrhal affections and skin diseases.

Aggravation

Heat of summer; hot weather.

Amelioration

Skin symptoms are better in cold weather (reverse of, Alum. and Petr.).

KALIUM BROMATUM

Potassium Bromide   **K. Br.**

Adapted to large persons inclined to obesity; acts better in children than in adults.

Loss of sensibility, fauces, larynx, urethra, entire body; staggering, uncertain gait; feels as if legs were all over sidewalk.

Nervous, restless; cannot sit still, must move about or keep occupied; *hands and fingers in constant motion; fidgety hands* (fidgety feet, Zinc.); twitching of fingers.

Fits of uncontrollable weeping and profound melancholic delusions.

Loss of memory; *forgets how to talk;* absentminded; has to be told the word before he could speak it (Anac.).

Depressed, low-spirited, anxious, "feel as if they would lose their minds."

Incoordination of muscles (Gels.); nervous weakness or paralysis of motion and numbness.

Restlessness and sleeplessness due to worry and grief, loss of property or reputation, from business embarrassments (Hyos.).

Night terrors of children (Kali-p.); grinding teeth in sleep, screams, moans, cries; horrible dreams, cannot be comforted by friends. Somnambulism (Sil.).

Spasms: From fright, anger or emotional causes in nervous plethoric persons; during parturition, teething, whooping cough, Bright's disease.

Epilepsy: Congenital, syphilitic, tubercular; usually a day or two before menses; at new moon; headache follows attack.

Cholera infantum, with reflex irritation of brain, before effusion; first stage of hydrocephaloid.

Daily colic in infants about 5 a.m. (at 4 p.m., Coloc., Lyc.).

Nervous cough during pregnancy; dry, hard, almost incessant, threatening abortion (Con.).

Stammering; slow, difficult speech (Bov., Stram.).

Acne: Simplex, indurata, rosacea; bluish-red, pustular, on face, chest, shoulders; leaves unsightly scars (Carb-an.); in young fleshy persons of gross habits.

Relationship

One of the antidotes for lead poisoning.

Often curative after Eugenia jambos in acne.

KALIUM CARBONICUM

Potassium Carbonate $K_2O_2CO_2$

For diseases of old people, dropsy and paralysis; with dark hair, lax fibre, inclined to obesity (Am-c., Graph.).

After loss of fluids or vitality, particularly in the anemic (Chin., Ph-ac., Phos., Psor.).

Pains *stitching, darting,* worse during rest and *lying*

on affected side (stitching, darting, better during rest and lying on painful side, Bry.).

Cannot bear to be touched; starts when touched ever so lightly, especially on the feet.

Great aversion to being alone (Ars., Bism., Lyc.; desires to be alone, Ign., Nux-v.).

Bag-like swelling between the upper eyelids and eyebrows.

Weak eyes; *after coition,* pollution, abortion, measles.

Stomach: Distended, sensitive; feels as if it would burst; excessive flatulency, everything she eats or drinks appears to be converted into gas (Iod.).

Nosebleed when *washing the face* in the morning (Am-c., Arn.).

Toothache *only when eating;* throbbing; < when touched by anything warm or cold.

Backache, sweating, weakness; after abortion, labor, metrorrhagia; when eating; while walking feels as if she must give up and lie down.

Cough: Dry, paroxysmal, loosens viscid mucus or pus which must be swallowed; spasmodic *with gagging or vomiting of ingesta;* hard, white or smoky masses fly from throat when coughing (Bad., Chel.).

Feels badly, week before menstruation; backache, before and during menses.

Labor pains insufficient; violent backache; wants the back pressed (Caust.).

Asthma, relieved when sitting up or bending forward or by rocking; worse from 2 to 4 a.m.

Persons suffering from ulceration of the lungs can scarcely get well without this anti-psoric – Hahnemann.

Difficult swallowing; sticking pain in pharynx as of a fish-bone (Hep., Nit-ac.); food easily gets into the windpipe; pain in back when swallowing.

Constipation: Stool large, difficult, with stitching, colic pains an hour or two before.

Heart: Tendency to fatty degeneration (Phos.); as if suspended by a thread (Lach.).

Very much inclined to take cold.

Relationship

Complementary: Carb-v.

Compare: Bry., Lyc., Nat-m., Nit-ac., Stann.

Follows well: After, Kali-s., Phos., Stann. in loose, rattling cough.

Will bring on the menses, when Nat-m., though apparently indicated, fails. — Hahnemann.

KALMIA LATIFOLIA

Mountain Laurel　　　　　　　　　　*Ericaceae*

Adapted to acute neuralgia, rheumatism, gouty complaints, especially when heart is involved as a sequele of rheumatism or gout.

In heart diseases that have developed from rheumatism, or alternate with it.

Pains sticking, darting, pressing, shooting *in a downward direction* (Cact.; upward, Led.); attended or succeeded by *numbness of affected part* (Acon., Cham., Plat.).

Severe stitching pain in right eye and orbit (left eye, Spig.); stiffness in muscles, pain < when turning the eyes (Spig.); begins at sunrise, < at noon and leaves at sunset (Nat-m.).

Rheumatism: Pains intense, change places suddenly, going from joint to joint; joint hot, red, swollen; worse from least movement.

Vertigo when stooping or looking down (Spig.).

Pulse slow, scarcely perceptible (35 or 40 per minute); pale face and cold extremities.

Relationship

Similar: To, Led., Rhod., Spig., in rheumatic affections and gout.

It follows Spig. well in heart disease.

KREOSOTUM

Kreosote   *A Distillation of Wood Tar*

Dark complexion, slight, lean, ill-developed, poorly nourished, *overgrown; very tall for her age* (Phos.).

Children: *Old looking, wrinkled* (Abrot.); scrofulous or psoric affections; rapid emaciation (Iod.); *post-climacteric diseases of women* (Lach.).

KREOSOTUM

Hemorrhage diathesis; small wounds bleed freely (Crot-h., Lach., Phos.); flow passive, in epistaxis, hemoptysis, hematuria; in typhoid, followed by great prostration; dark, oozing, after the extraction of a tooth (Ham.).

Roaring and humming in ears, with deafness, before and during menses.

Corrosive, fetid, ichorous discharges from mucous membranes; vitality greatly depressed.

Itching, so violent towards evening as to drive one almost wild (itching, without eruption, Dolichos).

Painful dentition; *teeth begin to decay as soon as they appear;* gums bluish-red, soft, spongy, bleeding, inflamed, scorbutic, ulcerated.

Vomiting: Of pregnancy, sweetish water with ptyalism; of cholera, during painful dentition; incessant with cadaverous stool; in malignant affections of stomach.

Severe headache before and during menses (Sep.).

Menses: Too early, profuse, protracted; pain during, but < after it; **flow on lying down,** cease on sitting or walking about; cold drinks relieve menstrual pains; *flow intermits,* at times almost ceasing, then commencing again (Sulph.).

Incontinence of urine; *can only urinate when lying;* copious, pale; urging, cannot get out of bed quick enough (Apis, Petros.); *during first sleep* (Sep.), from which child is roused with difficulty.

Smarting and burning during and after micturition (Sulph.).

Leucorrhea acrid, corrosive, offensive; *worse between periods* (Bov., Borx.); has the odor of green corn; stiffens like starch, stains the linen yellow.

Lochia: Dark, brown, lumpy, offensive, acrid; almost ceases, then freshens up again (Con., Sulph.).

Violent corrosive itching of pudenda and vagina.

Relationship

Kreosotum is followed well by Ars., Phos., Sulph., in cancer and disease of a malignant tendency.

Carb-v. and Kreos. are inimical.

Aggravation

In the open air, cold weather; when growing cold; from washing or bathing with cold water; rest, especially when lying.

Amelioration

Generally better from warmth.

LACHESIS

Surukuku Snake Poison   *Ophidia*

Persons of a less melancholy temperament, dark eyes, and a disposition to low spirits and indolence.

Women of choleric temperament, with freckles and red hair (Phos.).

Better adapted to thin and emaciated than to fleshy persons; to those who have been changed, both mentally and physically, by their illness.

Climacteric ailments; hemorrhoids, hemorrhages; **hot flushes and hot perspiration;** burning vertex headache, especially at or after the menopause (Sang., Sulph.).

Ailments from long lasting grief; sorrow, fright, vexation, jealousy or disappointed love (Aur., Ign., Phac.).

Women who have not recovered from the change of life "have never felt well since that time."

Left side principally affected; **diseases begin on the left and go to the right side** – left ovary, testicle, chest.

Great sensitiveness to touch; throat, stomach, abdomen; cannot bear bed-clothes or night-dress to touch throat or abdomen, not because sore or tender as in Apis or Bell., but clothes *cause an uneasiness,* make her nervous.

Intolerance of tight bands about neck or waist.

Extremes of heat and cold cause great debility.

Drunkards with congestive headaches and hemorrhoids; prone to erysipelas or apoplexy.

Headache: Pressing or bursting pain in temples < from motion, pressure, stooping, lying, after sleep; dreads to go to sleep because she wakens with such a headache.

Rush of blood to head; after alcohol; mental emotions; suppressed or irregular menses; at climaxis; left-sided apoplexy.

Weight and pressure on vertex (Sep.); like lead in occiput.

All symptoms, especially the mental, *worse after sleep, or the aggravation wakes him from sleep; sleeps into the aggravation,* unhappy, distressed, anxious, *sad < in morning on waking.*

Mental excitability; ecstasy with almost prophetic perceptions; with a vivid imagination; *great loquacity* (Agar., Stram.); wants to talk all the time; jumps from one idea to another; *one word often leads into another story.*

Constipation: Inactivity, stool lies in rectum, without urging; sensation of *constriction of sphincter* (Caust., Nit-ac.).

Menses **at regular time;** too short, scanty, feeble; *pains all relieved by the flow; always better during menses* (Zinc.).

Piles; with scanty menses; at climaxis; strangulated; with stitches shooting upward (Nit-ac.).

The least thing coming near mouth or nose interferes with breathing; wants to be fanned, *but slowly and at a distance* (rapidly, Carb-v.).

As soon as he falls asleep the breathing stops (Am-c., Grind., Lac-c., Op.).

Great physical and mental exhaustion; trembling in whole body, would constantly sink down from weakness; worse in the morning (Sulph., Tub.).

Epilepsy; comes on during sleep (Bufo); from loss of vital fluids; onanism, jealousy.

Hemorrhagic diathesis; small wounds bleed easily and profusely (Crot-h., Kreos., Phos.); blood dark, non-coagulable (Crot-h., Sec.).

Boils, carbuncles, ulcers with intense pain (Tarent.); malignant pustules; decubitus; *dark, bluish, purple appearance;* tend to malignancy.

Bad effects of poison wounds; post-mortem (Pyrog.). Sensation as of a ball rolling in the bladder.

Fever annually returning; paroxysm every spring (Carb-v., Sulph.); after suppression by quinine the previous autumn.

Fever: Typhoid, typhus; stupor or muttering delirium, sunken countenance, falling of lower jaw; tongue dry, black, *trembles,* is protruded with difficulty or *catches on the teeth* when protruding; conjunctiva yellow or orange color; perspiration cold, stains yellow, bloody (Lyc.).

Diphtheria and tonsillitis, *beginning on the left and extending to right side* (Lac-c., Sabad.); dark purple appearance (Naja); **< by hot drinks, after sleep;** *liquids more painful than solids* when swallowing (Bell., Bry., Ign.); prostration out of all proportion to appearance of throat.

Relationship

Complementary: Hep., Lyc., Nit-ac.

Incompatible: Acet-ac., Carb-ac.

In intermittent fever Nat-m. follows Lach. well when type changes.

Aggravation

After sleep; contact; extremes of temperature; acids; alcohol; cinchona; mercury; pressure or constriction; sun's rays; spring; summer.

LAC CANINUM

Dog's Milk

For nervous, restless, highly sensitive organisms.

Symptoms erratic, pains constantly flying from one part to another (Kali-bi., Puls.); *changing from side to side every few hours or days.*

Very forgetful, *absentminded;* makes purchases and walks away without them (Agn., Anac., Caust., Nat-m.).

In writing, uses too many words or not the right ones; omits final letter or letters in a word; cannot concentrate the mind to read or study; very nervous (Bov., Graph., Lach., Nat-c., Sep.).

Despondent, hopeless; thinks her disease incurable; has not a friend living; nothing worth living for; could weep at any moment (Cimic., Aur., Calc., Lach.).

Cross, irritable; child cries and screams all the time, especially at night (Jal., Nux-v., Psor.).

Fears to be alone (Kali-c.); of dying (Ars.); of becoming insane (Lil-t.); of falling down stairs (Borx.).

Chronic "blue" condition; everything seems so dark that it can grow no darker (Lyc., Puls.).

Attacks of rage, cursing and swearing at slightest provocation (Lil-t., Nit-ac.); intense ugliness; hateful.

Coryza, with discharge of thick, white mucus.

One nostril stuffed up, the other free and discharging; these conditions alternate; discharge acrid, nose and lip raw (All-c., Arum-t.).

Diphtheria and tonsillitis; symptoms *change repeatedly from side to side.*

Sore throats and cough are apt to *begin and end with menstruation;* yellow or white patches; pains shoot to ear.

Throat: Sensitive to touch externally (Lach.); < by empty swallowing (Ign.); constant inclination to swallow, *painful,* almost impossible (Merc.); *pains extend to ears* (Hep., Kali-bi.); begins on left side (Lach.).

Shining, glazed appearance of diphtheritic deposit, chancres and ulcers.

Very hungry, cannot eat enough to satisfy; as hungry after eating as before (Casc., Calc., Cina, Lyc., Stront.).

Sinking at epigastrium; *faintness in stomach.*

Menses: Too early; too profuse; flow in gushes, bright red, viscid and stringy (dark, black, stringy, Croc.); breasts swollen, painful, sensitive before and during (Con.).

Discharge of flatus from vagina (Brom., Lyc., Nux-m., Sang.).

Breasts: Inflamed, painful; < by least jar and towards evening; *must hold them firmly when going up or down stairs* (Bry.).

Serviceable in almost all cases when it is required to dry up milk (Asaf.; to bring back or increase it, Lac-d.).

Sensation as if breath would leave her when lying down; must get up and walk (Am-c., Grind., Lach.).

Loss of milk while nursing without any known cause (Asaf.).

Palpitation violent when lying on left side > turning on right (Tab.).

Sexual organs easily excited, from touch, pressure on sitting, or friction by walking (Cinnm., Coff., Murx., Plat.).

When walking, seems to be walking on air; when lying, does not seem to touch the bed (Asar.).

Backache: Intense, unbearable, across super-sacral region, extending to right natis and right sciatic nerve; < by rest and on first moving (Rhus-t.); spine aches from base of brain to coccyx, *very sensitive to touch or pressure* (Chinin-s., Phos., Zinc.).

Relationship

Similar: To, Apis, Con., Murx., Lach., Kali-bi., Puls., Sep., Sulph.

It generally acts best in single dose.

Probably no remedy in the materia medica presents a more valuable pathogenesis in symptoms of the throat, or one that will better repay a careful study.

Like Lachesis, this remedy has met with the most violent opposition form prejudice and ignorance, which its wonderful therapeutic powers have slowly, yet surely, overcome. It was successfully used by Dioscorides, Pliny, and Sextus in ancient times, and revived in New York by Reisig, Bayard and Swan in the successful treatment of diphtheria. Reisig was the first to potentize it.

LAC DEFLORATUM

Skimmed Milk

The successful treatment of diabetes and Bright's disease with skimmed milk, by Donkin, was the hint which led Dr. Swan to potentize and prove it. Every symptom here given has been verified in the cure of the sick.

Diseases with faulty and defective nutrition with reflex affections of nervous centers.

Despondent; does not care to live; has no fear of death but it sure he is going to die.

American sick headache: Begins in forehead, extending to occiput, in morning, on rising (Bry.); *intense throbbing,* with nausea, vomiting, *blindness* and obstinate constipation (Epig., Iris, Sang.); < noise, light, motion (Mag-m., Sil.), during menses (Kreos., Sep.); great prostration; > pressure, by bandaging head tightly (Arg-n., Puls.); copious, pale urine.

Globus hystericus: Sensation of a large ball rising from stomach to throat, causing sense of suffocation (Asaf., Kalm.).

Vomiting: Incessant, no relation to eating; first of undigested food, intensely acid, then of bitter water; *of pregnancy* (Lac-ac., Psor.).

Constipation: With ineffectual urging (Anac., Nux-v.); feces dry and hard (Bry., Sulph.); *stool large, hard, great straining, lacerating anus;* **painful, extorting cries.**

A woman had taken 10 or 12 enemas daily, often

passed 4 or 5 weeks without an evacuation, cured constipation of 15 years' standing.

Menses: Delayed; suppressed by *putting hands in cold water* (Con.); *drinking a glass of milk will promptly suppress flow until next period* (compare, Phos.).

Great restlessness, extreme and protracted suffering from *loss of sleep* (Cocc., Nit-ac.).

Feels completely exhausted, whether she does anything or not; great fatigue when walking.

Sensation: As if cold air was blowing on her, even while covered up; as if sheets were damp.

Dropsy: From organic heart disease; from chronic liver complaint; far advanced albuminuria; following intermittent fever.

Obesity; fatty degeneration.

LEDUM PALUSTRE

Marsh Tea *Ericaceae*

Adapted to the rheumatic, gouty diathesis; constitutions abused by alcohol (Colch.).

Hemorrhage into anterior chamber after iridectomy.

Contusions of eye and lids, especially if much extravasation of blood; ecchymosis of lids and conjunctiva.

Rheumatism or gout; *beings in lower limbs and ascends*

(descends, Kalm.); especially if brought to a low asthenic condition by abuse of Colchicum; joints become the seat of nodosities and "gout stones" which are painful; acute and chronic arthritis.

Affects left shoulder and right hip joint (Agar., Ant-t., Stram.).

Emaciation of affected parts (Graph.).

Pains are sticking, tearing, throbbing; rheumatic pains are < by motion; < at night, by warmth of *bed and bed covering* (Merc.); > *only when holding feet in ice-water* (Sec.).

Complaints of people who are *cold all the time; always feel cold and chilly;* lack of animal or vital heat (Sep., Sil.); the wounded parts especially are *cold to touch.*

Parts cold to touch, but not cold subjectively to patient.

In some affections, warmth of bed intolerable on account of heat and burning of limbs.

Swelling: Of feet, up to knees; of ankle with unbearable pain when walking, as from a sprain or false step; ball of great toe swollen, painful; in heels as if bruised.

Intense itching of feet and ankles, < from scratching warmth of bed (Puls., Rhus-t.).

Easy spraining of ankles and feet (Carb-an.).

Punctured wounds by sharp, pointed instruments, as awls, nails (Hyper.); rat bites, stings of insects, especially mosquitoes.

Red pimples or tubercles *on forehead and cheeks,* as in brandy drinkers, stinging when touched.

Long-remaining *discoloration after injuries;* "black and blue" places *become green.*

Relationship

Compare: Arn., Crot-t., Ham., Bell-p., Ruta, in traumatism; Con. in long-lasting effects of injuries.

LILIUM TIGRINUM

Tiger Lily *Liliaceae*

Affects principally the left side of the body (Lach., Thuj.).

Tormented about her salvation (Lyc., Sulph., Verat.), with ovarian or uterine complaints; consolation <.

Wild, crazy feeling on vertex; confused ideas.

Profound depression of spirits, can hardly avoid weeping; is very timid, fearful and weeps much; indifferent about what is being done for her.

Anxious: About the disease; fears the symptoms indicate an organic affection; marked in both sexes.

Disposed to curse, strike, to think obscene things (Anac., Lac-c.); alternates with uterine irritation.

Listless, yet cannot sit still; restless, yet does not want to walk; *must keep busy to repress sexual desire.*

Desire to do something, hurried manner, yet has no ambition; *aimless, hurried motion* (Arg-n.).

Fears: Being alone, insanity, heart disease; fears she is incurable; some impending calamity or disease.

Headaches and mental ailments depending on uterine irritation or displacements. Menstrual irregularities and irritable heart.

Cannot walk on uneven ground.

Pains in small spots; constantly shifting (Kali-bi.).

Frequent urging to urinate; if desire is not attended to, sensation of congestion in chest.

Bearing-down sensation; in abdomen and pelvis, as though all organs would escape (Lac-c., Murx., Sep.); < supporting vulva with hand; with palpitation.

Menses: Early, scanty, dark, offensive; **flow only when moving about;** cease to flow when she ceases to walk (Caust.; on lying down, Kreos., Mag-c.).

Sensation as if heart was *grasped in a vise* (Cact.); as if blood had all gone to the heart; feels full to bursting; inability to walk erect.

Pulsations over whole body, and full, distended feeling as if blood would burst through the vessel (Aesc.).

Palpitation: Fluttering; faint, hurried, anxious sensation about apex; sharp pain in left chest awakens at night; irregular pulse; extremities cold and covered with cold sweat; < after eating, lying on either side (on left side, Lach.).

Rapid heart-beat, 150 to 170 per minute.

Constant desire to defecate and urinate (with prolapsus), from pressure in rectum.

Weak and atonic condition of ovaries, uterus and pelvic tissues, resulting in anteversion, retroversion, sub-involution (Helon., Sep.); slow recovery after labor; nearly always with constipation, from inactivity.

Relationship

Compare: Agar., Cact., Cimic., Helon., Murx., Nat-p., Plat., Sep., Spig., Tarent.

LOBELIA INFLATA

Indian Tobacco *Lobeliaceae*

Best adapted to persons of light hair, blue eyes, fair complexion; inclined to be fleshy.

Gastric derangements, *extreme nausea and vomiting*; morning sickness; spasmodic asthma; *pertussis, with dyspnea threatening suffocation.*

Headache: Gastric, with nausea, vomiting and great prostration; following intoxication; < afternoon until midnight; sudden pallor with profuse sweat (Tab.); < by tobacco or tobacco smoke.

Vomiting: *Face bathed with cold sweat;* of pregnancy, *profuse salivation* (Lac-c.; at night, Merc.); **chronic with good appetite, with nausea, profuse sweat and marked prostration.**

Faintness, weakness and an indescribable feeling at epigastrium, from excessive use of tea or tobacco.

Urine: Of a deep orange red color; copious red sediment.

Dyspnea: From constriction of middle of chest; < with every labor pain, seems to neutralize the pains; < by exposure to cold or slightest exertion, going up or down stairs (Ip.).

Sensation of congestion, pressure or weight in chest as if blood from extremities was filling it, > *by rapid walking*.

Sensation as if heart would stand still; deep-seated pain at base (at apex, Lil-t.).

Sacrum: **Extreme sensitiveness;** *cannot bear the slightest touch, even of a soft pillow*; sits leaning forward to avoid contact with clothes.

Relationship

Compare: Ant-t., Ars., Ip., Tab., Verat.

Aggravation

Slightest motion; touch, cold.

Amelioration

Chest pain by walking rapidly.

For the bad effects of drunkenness in people with light hair, blue or grey eyes, florid complexion, corpulent, Lobelia bears the same relation that Nux vomica does to persons of the opposite temperament.

LYCOPODIUM CLAVATUM

Wolf's Foot; Club Moss   *Lycopodiaceae*

For persons intellectually keen, but physically weak; upper part of body emaciated, lower part semi-dropical; predisposed to lung and hepatic affections (Calc., Phos., Sulph.); especially in extremes of life, children and old people.

Deep-seated, progressive, chronic diseases.

Pains: Aching-pressure, drawing; chiefly right-sided, < **four to eight p.m.**

Affects right side, or pain goes from right to left, throat, chest, abdomen, liver, ovaries.

Children, weak, emaciated; with well developed head but puny, sickly bodies.

Baby cries all day, sleeps all night (Jal., Psor.).

Ailments from fright, anger, mortification, or vexation with reserved displeasure (Staph.).

Avaricious, greedy, miserly, malicious, pusillanimous.

Irritable; peevish and cross on waking; ugly, kick and scream; easily angered; cannot endure opposition or contradiction; seeks disputes; is beside himself.

Weeps all day, cannot calm herself; very sensitive, even cries when thanked.

Dread of men; of solitude, irritable and melancholy; fear of being alone (Bism., Kali-c., Lil-t.).

LYCOPODIUM CLAVATUM

Complexion pale, dirty; unhealthy; sallow, with deep furrows, looks older than he is; *fan-like motion of alae nasi* (Ant-t.).

Catarrh: Dry nose *stopped at night*, must breathe through the mouth (Am-c., Nux-v., Samb.); snuffles, child starts from sleep rubbing its nose; of root of nose and frontal sinuses; crusts and elastic plugs (Kali-bi., Teucr.).

Diphtheria: Fauces brownish-red, deposit spreads *from right tonsil to left*, or descends from nose to right tonsils; < after sleep and **from cold drinks** (from warm drinks, Lach.).

Everything tastes sour; eructations, heartburn, waterbrash, sour vomiting (between chill and heat).

Canine hunger; the more he eats, the more he craves; head aches if he does not eat.

Gastric affections: **Excessive accumulation of flatulence;** constant sensation of satiety; good appetite, but **a few mouthfuls fill up to the throat,** and *he feels bloated;* fermentation in abdomen, with *loud grumbling, croaking,* especially lower abdomen (upper abdomen, Carb-v.; entire abdomen, Chin.); fullness, not relieved by belching (Chin.).

Constipation: Since puberty; since last confinement; when away from home; of infants; with ineffectual urging, rectum contracts and protrudes during stool, developing piles.

Red sand in urine, on child's diaper (Phos.); *child cries before urinating* (Borx.); pain in back, relieved by urinating; renal colic, right side (left side, Berb.).

Impotence: Of young men, from onanism or sexual excess; penis small, cold, relaxed; *old men, with strong desire but imperfect erections;* falls asleep during an embrace; premature emission.

Dryness of vagina; burning in, during and after coition (Lyss.); physometra.

Discharge of blood from genitals during every stool.

Fetus appears to be turning somersaults.

Hernia: Right sided, has cured many cases especially in children.

Pneumonia; neglected or maltreated, base of right lung involved especially; to hasten absorption or expectoration.

Cough deep, hollow, even raising mucus in large quantities affords little relief.

One foot hot and the other cold (Chin., Dig., Ip.).

Waking at night feeling hungry (Cina, Psor.).

Relationship

Complementary: Iodine.

Bad effects: Of onions, bread; wine, spirituous liquors; tobacco smoking and chewing (Ars.).

Follows well: After, Calc., Carb-v., Lach., Sulph.

It is rarely advisable to begin the treatment of a chronic disease with Lyc. unless clearly indicated; it is better to give first another anti-psoric.

Lyc. is a deep-seated, long-acting remedy, and should rarely be repeated after improvement begins.

Aggravation

Nearly all diseases from 4 to 8 p.m. (Hell.; from 4 to 9 p.m., Coloc., Mag-p.).

Amelioration

Warm foods and drinks; from uncovering the head; loosening the garments.

LYSSINUM*

The Saliva of a Rabid Dog *A Nosode*

The sight or sound of running water or pouring water aggravates all complaints.

Lyssophobia, fear of becoming mad.

Bluish discoloration of wounds (Lach.).

Complaints resulting from abnormal sexual desire (from abstinence, Con.).

Mental emotion or mortifying news always makes him worse.

Cannot bear heat of sun (Gels., Glon., Lach., Nat-m.).

Convulsions: From dazzling or reflected light from water or mirror (Stram.); from even thinking of fluids of any kind; from slightest touch or current of air.

---

* Zincum suggests Lyssin as a substitute for Hydrophobinum Encyclopaedia, Vol. iii, p. 472.

Headache: From bites of dogs, whether rabid or not; chronic, from mental emotion or exertion; < *by noise of running water or bright light.*

Saliva: Tough, ropy, viscid, frothy in mouth and throat, with constant spitting (Hydr.).

Sore throat, constant desire to swallow (Lac-c., Merc.).

Difficulty in swallowing, even spasm of esophagus from swallowing liquids; gagging when swallowing water.

Constant desire to urinate on *seeing running water* (Canth., Sulph.); urine scanty, cloudy, contains sugar.

Prolapsus uteri; many cases of years' standing cured.

Sensitiveness of vagina, rendering coition, painful.

Relationship

Compare: Bell., Canth., Hyos., Stram., in hydrophobia.

Aggravation

Sight or sound of water; bright, dazzling light (Stram.); carriage riding (Cocc.; better from, Nit-ac.).

MAGNESIUM CARBONICUM

Carbonate of Magnesia $MgCO_3\ 3H_2O$

For persons, especially children, of irritable disposition, nervous temperament (Cham.); lax fibre;

sour smell of whole body (Rheum).

The whole body feels tired and painful, especially the legs and feet; aching, restless.

Spasmodic affections of stomach and intestines (Coloc., Mag-p.), increased secretions from mucous membranes.

Unrefreshing sleep, more tired on rising than when retiring (Bry., Con., Hep., Op., Sulph.).

Inordinate *craving for meat* in children of tuberculous parentage.

Heartburn: *Sour,* belching, eructations, taste and vomiting; of *pregnancy.*

Pains: Neuralgic, lightning-like, < left side (Coloc.); insupportable during repose, must get up and walk (Rhus-t.); toothache, during *pregnancy < at night.*

Pain on vertex as if the hair were pulled (Kali-n., Phos.).

Menses: Preceded by sore throat (Lac-c.), labor-like pain, cutting colic, backache, weakness, chilliness; flows **only at night or when lying,** ceases when walking (Am-m., Kreos.; reverse of Lil-t.); acrid, dark, pitch-like; difficult to wash off (Med.).

Diarrhea: Preceded by cutting, doubling-up colic; occurs regularly every three weeks; *stools green, frothy,* **like scum on a frog-pond;** white, tallow-like masses are found floating in stool; the milk *passes undigested in nursing children.*

When crude magnesia has been taken to "sweeten the stomach"; if the symptoms corresponds, the potentized remedy will often relieve.

Relationship

Complementary: To, Chamomilla.

Aggravation

Change of temperature; *every three weeks*; rest; milk, during menses.

Amelioration

Warm air, but worse in warmth of bed (Led., Merc. — better in warmth of bed, Ars.).

MAGNESIUM MURIATICUM

Chloride of Magnesia   *MgCl*

Especially adapted to diseases of women; spasmodic and hysterical complaints, complicated with uterine diseases; who have suffered for years from attacks of indigestion or biliousness.

Children: During difficult dentition **are unable to digest milk;** it causes pain in stomach and passes undigested; puny, rachitic, who crave sweets.

Great sensitiveness to noise (Ign., Nux-v., Ther.).

Headache: Every six weeks, in forehead and around the eyes; as if it would burst; < from motion and in open air; > from lying down, *strong pressure* (Puls.), and wrapping up warmly (Sil., Stront.).

Great tendency of head to sweat (Calc., Sanic., Sil.).

Continual rising of white froth into the mouth.

Eructations, tasting like rotten eggs, like onions (breath smells of onions, Sinap.).

Toothache; unbearable when food touches the teeth.

Pressing pain in liver, when walking and touching it, liver hard, enlarged, < lying on right side (Merc., Kali-c.).

Constipation: Stool hard, scanty, large, knotty, like sheep's dung; difficult to pass; **crumbling at verge of anus** (Am-m., Nat-m.); *of infants during dentition.*

Urine: Pale, yellow, can only be passed by bearing down with abdominal muscles; weakness of bladder.

Menses with great excitement at every period; flow black, clotted; spasms and pains < in back when walking, extend into thighs; metrorrhagia, < at night in bed, causing hysteria (Caul., Cimic.).

Leucorrhea: After exercise; with every stool; with uterine spasm; followed by metrorrhagia; two weeks after menses for three or four days. (Bar-c., Bov., Con.).

Palpitation and cardiac pains while sitting, < by moving about (compare, Gels.).

Relationship

Compare: Cham. in the disease of children.

MAGNESIUM PHOSPHORICUM

Is best adapted to thin, emaciated persons of a highly nervous organization; dark complexion.

Affections of *right side of body*; head, ear, face, chest, ovary, sciatic nerve (Bell., Bry., Chel., Kali-c., Lyc., Podo.).

Pains: Sharp, cutting, stabbing; shooting, stitching; *lightning-like in coming and going* (Bell.); intermittent paroxysm becoming almost unbearable, driving patient to frenzy; rapidly changing place (Lac-c., Puls.), with a constricting sensation (Cact., Iod., Sulph.), **cramping**, in neuralgic affections of stomach, abdomen and pelvis (Caul., Coloc.).

Great dread: Of cold air; **of uncovering;** of touching affected part; of cold bathing or washing; of moving.

Languid, tired, exhausted; unable to sit up.

Complaints from standing in cold water or working in cold clay (Calc.).

Ailments of teething children; *spasms during dentition, no fever* (with fever, hot head and skin, Bell.).

Headache: Begins in occiput and extends over head (Sang., Sil.); of school girls; face red, flushed; from mental emotion, exertion or hard study; < 10 to 11 a.m. or 4 to 5 p.m.; > by pressure and external heat.

Neuralgia: Of face, supra or infra-orbital; right side; intermittent, darting, cutting; < by touch, cold air, pressure; > by external heat.

Toothache: At night; rapidly shifting; < eating, drinking, especially cold things; > by heat (> by cold, Bry., Coff., Ferr-p.).

Spasms or cramp of stomach, with clean tongue, as if a band was drawn tightly around the body.

Colic: Flatulent, forcing patient to bend double; > by heat, rubbing and hard pressure (Coloc., Plb.); of horses and cows when Colocynthis fails to >.

Menses: Early; flow dark, stringy; pains < before, > when flow begins (Lach., Zinc.); pains darting, like lightning, shooting, < right side, > by heat and bending double; vaginismus.

Enuresis: Nocturnal; from nervous irritation; urine, pale, copious; *after catheterization*.

Cramps: Of extremities; during pregnancy; of *writers*, piano or violin players.

Relationship

Compare: Bell., Caul., Coloc., Lyc., Lac-c., Puls.; Cham. is its vegetable analogue.

Sometimes acts best when given in hot water.

Aggravation

Cold air; a draft of cold air or cold wind; cold bathing or washing; motion; touch.

Amelioration

Bending double; heat; warmth; pressure (burning pain > by heat, Ars.).

MEDORRHINUM

The Gonorrheal Virus *A Nosode*

For the constitutional effects of maltreated and suppressed gonorrhea, when the best selected remedy fails to relieve or permanently improve.

For persons suffering from gout, rheumatism, neuralgia and diseases of the spinal cord and its membranes—even organic lesions ending in paralysis—which can be traced to a sycotic origin.

For women, with chronic ovaritis, salpingitis, pelvic cellulitis, fibroids, cysts, and other morbid growths of the uterus and ovaries, especially if symptoms point to malignancy with or without sycotic origin.

For scirrhus, carcinoma or cancer; either acute or chronic in development, when the symptoms correspond and a history of sycosis can be traced.

Bears the same relation to deep-seated sycotic chronic affections of spinal and sympathetic nervous system, that Psorinum does to deep-seated affections of skin and mucous membranes.

Children, pale, rachitic; dwarfed and stunted in growth (Bar-c.); mentally, dull and weak.

Great heat and soreness, with enlargement of lymphatic glands all over body.

Consumptive languor; fatigue; great general depression of vitality.

Pains: Arthritic, rheumatic, a sequel of suppressed gonorrhea (Daph., Clem.); constricting, seem to tighten the whole body (Cact.); sore all over, as if bruised (Arn., Eup-per.).

Trembling all over (subjective); intense nervousness and profound exhaustion.

State of collapse, wants to be fanned all the time (Carb-v.); craves fresh air; skin cold, yet throws off the covers (Camph., Sec.); cold and bathed with cold perspiration (Verat.).

Mind: Weakness of memory; cannot remember names, words or initial letters; has to ask name of most intimate friend; even forgets his own name.

Cannot spell correctly; wonders how a well-known name is spelled.

Constantly loses the thread of conversation.

Great difficulty in stating her symptoms, question has to be repeated as she loses herself.

Cannot speak without weeping.

Anticipates death; always anticipating, feels matters most sensitively before they occur and generally correctly.

Irritated at trifles; cross during the day, exhilarated at night.

Very impatient; peevish.

Anxious, nervous, extremely sensitive; starts at the least sound.

Time passes too slowly (Alum., Arg-n., Cann-i.).

Is in a great hurry; when doing anything is in such a hurry she gets fatigued.

MEDORRHINUM

Many symptoms are < when thinking of them (pains return as soon as he thinks about them, Ox-ac.).

Head: Intense burning pain in brain, < in cerebellum; extends down spine.

Head feels heavy and is drawn backwards.

Sensation of tightness and contraction; extends down whole length of spine.

Headache and diarrhea from jarring of cars.

Throat: Sensation as if she had taken a severe cold, with distressing aching in bones; throat sore and swollen, deglutition of either liquids or solids impossible (Merc.).

Throat constantly filled with thick, gray or bloody mucus from posterior nates (Hydr.).

Appetite: Ravenous hunger immediately after eating (Chin., Lyc., Psor.).

Constant thirst, even dreams she is drinking.

Insatiate craving: For liquor, which, before she hated (Asar.); for salt (Calc., Nat-m.); for sweets (Sulph.); for ale, ice, acids, oranges, green fruit.

Bowels: Stools: Tenacious, clay-like, sluggish, cannot strain from a sensation of prolapse of rectum (Alum.).

Constriction and inertia of bowels with ball-like stools (Lach.).

Can only pass stool by leaning very far back; very painful as if there was a lump on posterior surface of sphincter; so painful as to cause tears.

Sharp, needle-like pains in rectum.

Oozing of moisture from anus, fetid odor of fish brine (Caust., Hep.).

Urinary Organs: Severe pain (backache) in renal region, > by profuse urination (Lyc.).

Renal colic; intense pain in ureters, with sensation of passing of calculus (Berb., Lyc., Oci.); craving for ice.

Nocturnal enuresis: Passes enormous quantity of ammoniacal, high-colored urine in bed every night; < by over-work or over-play, extremes of heat or cold, when the best selected remedy fails; with a history of sycosis.

Painful tenesmus of bladder and bowels when urinating.

Sexual Organs: Menses: Profuse, very dark, clotted; stains difficult to wash out (Mag-c.).

Metrorrhagia: At climacteric; profuse for weeks, flow dark, clotted, offensive; in gushes, on moving; with malignant disease of uterus.

Intense menstrual colic with drawing up of knees and terrible bearing down labor-like pains; must press feet against support, as in labor.

Intense pruritus of labia and vagina < by thinking of it.

Breasts and nipples sore and sensitive to touch.

Breasts cold as ice to touch, especially the nipples, rest of body warm (during menses).

Respiratory Organs: Asthma: Choking caused by a weakness or spasm of epiglottis; larynx stopped so that no air could enter, only > by lying on face and protruding tongue.

Soreness of larynx as if ulcerated.

Dyspnea and sense of constriction; can inhale with ease, but no power to exhale (Samb.).

Cough: Dry, incessant, severe; painful, as if mucous membrane was torn from larynx; deep, hollow, like coughing in a barrel; < at night, from sweets, on lying down; > by lying on stomach.

Sputa: Albuminous, frothy; small, green, bitter balls; viscid, difficult to raise.

Incipient consumption; severe pains in middle lobes.

Back and Extremities: Pain in back between scapulae; whole length of spine sore to touch (Chinin-s.).

Intense burning heat, beginning in nape of neck and extending down spine, with a contractive stiffness, < by stretching.

Rheumatism at top of shoulder and arm; pains extend to fingers, > by motion (right, Sang.; left, Ferr.).

Lumbar vertebrae painful and sensitive to touch.

Pain in sacrum, coccyx, and back of hips running around and down limbs.

Pain in legs, from hips to knees; only when walking.

Heaviness of legs, feel like lead; walking very difficult, legs are so heavy; legs give way.

Lower limbs ache all night, preventing sleep.

Intense restless and fidgety legs and feet (Zinc.).

Terrible burning in legs and arms during an electrical storm.

Aching in legs, with inability to keep them still in bed, < when giving up control of himself, when relaxing, in trying to sleep.

Coldness of legs and feet; of hands and forearms.

Drawing, contracting sensation in hamstrings and ankles; cramps in calves and soles (Cupr.).

Ankles turn easily when walking (Carb-an., Led.).

Burning of hands and feet, wants them covered and fanned (Lach., Sulph.).

Almost entire loss of nervous force in legs and arms; exhausted by slightest effort.

Painful stiffness of every joint in body.

Deformity of finger joints; *large, puffy knuckles*; swelling and painful stiffness of ankles; great tenderness of heels and balls of feet; swellings of all joints, were puffy, like windgalls.

Relationship

Compare: Ip., dry cough; Camph., Sec., Tab., Verat., in collapse; Pic-ac., Gels., inability to walk; Aloe, Sulph., morning diarrhea.

The burning feet of Sulphur and restless fidgety legs and feet of Zinc. are both found at the same time in Medorrhinum.

Aggravation

When thinking of it (Helon., Ox-ac.); heat, covering;

stretching; thunderstorm; least movement; sweets; from daylight to sunset (reverse of Syph.).

Amelioration

At the seashore (reverse of Nat-m.); lying on stomach; damp weather (Caust., Nux-v.).

MELILOTUS ALBA

Sweet Clover *Leguminosae*

Congestions, *relieved by hemorrhage.*

Engorgement of blood vessels in any part or organ.

Violent congestive or nervous headaches; *epistaxis affords relief* (Bufo, Ferr-p., Mag-s.).

Convulsions: Of nervous children during dentition (Bell.); infantile spasms, eclampsia, epilepsy.

Religious melancholy with an intensely red face; insanity, in early stages, to relieve brain from pressure and irritation.

Nosebleed preceded by **intense redness, flushing of face and throbbing of carotids** (Bell.); with general relief.

Very red face precedes hemorrhage from every organ.

Constipation: Difficult, painful, constriction in anus; throbbing, fulness; no desire until there is a large ammuculation (Alum.).

Relationship

Compare: Aml-ns., Ant-c. in epistaxis after headache, but does not relieve; Bell., Glon., Sang., in congestive headache, red face, hot head, etc.

Aggravation

Approach of a storm; rainy, changeable weather.

MENYANTHES TRIFOLIATA

Buck Bean *Gentianaceae*

Complaints from abuse of cinchona and quinine.

Fevers, in which the cold stage predominates; coldness felt most acutely in abdomen and legs.

Headache: *Pressing in vertex* from above downwards, > *during hard pressure with hand* (Verat.); as of a *heavy weight* pressing upon the head at every step (Cact., Glon., Lach.); < ascending (Calc.); often with icy coldness of hands and feet (Calc., Sep.).

Anxiety about the heart as if some evil was impending.

Tension: In root of nose; in arms, hands, fingers; in skin, as if several sizes too small and was crowded into it by force.

Relationship

Compare: Cact., Calc., Gels., Sep., Mag-m., Par.

Follow well: Caps., Lach., Lyc., Puls., Rhus-t., Verat.

Aggravation

During rest; lying down.

Amelioration

Pressure on affected part.

MERCURIUS

Quicksilver　　　　　　　　　　*The Element*

Best adapted for light-haired persons; skin and muscles lax.

In bone diseases, **pains worse at night;** glandular swellings with or without suppuration. But especially if suppuration be too profuse (Hep., Sil.).

Cold swellings; abscesses, slow to suppurate.

Profuse perspiration attends nearly every complaint, but *does not relieve;* may even increase the suffering (profuse perspiration relieves, Nat-m., Psor., Verat.).

Great weakness and trembling from least exertion.

Breath and body smell foul (Psor.).

Hurried and rapid talking (Hep.).

Catarrh: With much sneezing; fluent, acrid, corrosive; nostrils raw, ulcerated; yellow-green, fetid, pus-like; nasal bones swollen; < at night and from *damp weather*.

Toothache: Pulsating, tearing, lacerating, shooting into face or ears; < in damp weather or evening air, warmth of bed, from cold or warm things; > from rubbing the cheek.

Crowns of teeth decay, roots remain (crowns intact, roots decay, Mez.).

Ptyalism; tenacious, soapy, stringy, profuse, *fetid coppery, metallic-tasting saliva.*

Tongue: **Large, flabby, shows imprint of teeth** (Chel., Podo., Rhus-t.); painful, with ulcers; red or white.

Intense thirst although the tongue looks moist and the saliva is profuse (dry mouth, but no thirst, Puls.).

Mumps, diphtheria, tonsillitis with *profuse offensive saliva;* tongue large, flabby with imprint of teeth; mapped tongue (Lach., Nat-m., Tarax.).

Diphtheria: Tonsils inflamed, uvula swollen, elongated, *constant desire to swallow;* membrane thick, gray, shred-like borders adherent or free.

Dysentery: **Stool slimy, bloody,** *with colic and fainting;* great tenesmus *during and* **after, not** > by stool, followed by chilliness and a "cannot finish" sensation. *The more blood,* the better indicated.

Quantity of urine voided is larger than the amount of water drunk; frequent urging to urinate.

Nocturnal emissions stained with blood (Led., Sars.).

Leucorrhea: Acrid, burning, *itching with rawness; always worse at night;* pruritus, < from contact of urine which must be washed off (Sulph.).

Morning sickness; profuse salivation, wets the pillow in sleep (Lac-ac.).

Mammae painful, as if they would ulcerate at *every menstrual period* (Con., Lac-c.); milk in breasts instead of the menses.

Cough: Dry, fatiguing, racking; in two paroxysms, *worse at night* and from *warmth of bed;* with utter inability to lie on right side.

Affects lower lobe of right lung; stitches through to back (Chel., Kali-c.).

Suppuration of lungs, after hemorrhages of pneumonia (Kali-c.).

Ulcers on the gums, tongue, throat, inside of the cheek, with profuse salivation; irregular in shape, edges undefined; have a dirty, unhealthy look; lardaceous base surrounded with a dark halo; apt to run together (syphilitic ulcers are circular, attack the posterior parts of mouth, throat and have well defined edges, are surrounded with a coppery hue, and do not extend from their primary seat).

Trembling extremities, especially hands; paralysis agitans.

Relationship

Follows well: After, Bell., Hep., Lach., Sulph., but should not be given before or after Silicea.

If given in low (weak) potencies hastens rather than aborts suppuration.

The bad effects of Merc. are antidoted by Aur., Hep., Lach., Mez., Nit-ac., Sulph., and by a strong (high) potency of Merc., when the symptoms corresponds.

Compare: Mezereum, its vegetable analogue, for bad effects of large doses or of too frequent repetition.

Ailments from sugar, insect stings, vapors of arsenic or copper. Diseases occurring in winter.

Aggravation

At night; wet, damp weather (Rhus-t.); in autumn, warm days and cold, damp nights; lying on right side; perspiring.

Mercury is < by heat of, but > by rest in, bed.

Arsenic is > by heat of, but < by rest in, bed.

MERCURIUS BINIODATUS

Biniodide of Mercury MgI_2

Diphtheritic and glandular affections *of left side;* fauces dark red; solids or liquids painful when swallowing; exudation slight, easily detached; cases attending epidemic scarlet fever, ulcers on fauces or tonsils; glands enlarged; greenish tough lumps from pharynx or posterior nares.

Tubercular pharyngitis.

MERCURIUS CORROSIVUS

Corrosive Sublimate $HgCl_2$

Diseases of men, syphilitic; ulcers, with corroding, acrid pus; Bright's disease.

Dysentery and summer complaints of intestinal canal, occurring from May to November.

Tenesmus: Of rectum, *not > by stool* (< by stool, Nux-v.); incessant, persistent; stool hot, *scanty, bloody, slimy, offensive;* shreds of mucous membrane and terrible cutting, colicky pains.

Tenesmus: Of bladder, with intense burning in urethra; urine hot, burning, scanty or suppressed; in drops with great pain; bloody, brown, brick-dust sediment; albuminous.

Gonorrhea: Second stage, *greenish discharge*, < at night; great burning and tenesmus.

MERCURIUS CYANATUS

Cyanide of Mercury $Hg\,(CN_2)$

Malignant diphtheria with *intense redness of fauces* and great difficulty of swallowing; pseudo-membranous formation extends all over fauces and down throat; putrid, gangrenous diphtheria, with phagedenic ulceration; membranous croup.

Great weakness; extreme prostration; cannot stand up from weakness.

When it corresponds to the genus epidemicus, like every other remedy, is effective as a prophylactic.

MERCURIUS DULCIS

Calomel Hg_2Cl_2

Catarrhal affections of mucous membranes, especially of the eye and ear.

Catarrhal inflammation of middle ear (Kali-m.).

Eustachian tube closed; catarrhal deafness and otorrhea in psoric children; deafness of old age (Kali-m.).

Acute affections of prostate after maltreated stricture.

Deafness and catarrhal affections of nares, throat, and pharynx, from mercurial amalgam fillings.

Diarrhea: Of children; stools grass-green; like chopped eggs; profuse, causing soreness of anus.

MERCURIUS PROTO-IODATUS

Iodide of Mercury Hg_2I_2

Diphtheritic and throat affections where the cervical and parotid glands are enormously swollen; membrane begins on or is < on right side; < by warm drinks, and empty swallowing (Lach.).

Tongue: **Thick, yellow coating at base** (Kali-bi.; *golden yellow* coating at base, Nat-p.; dirty or greenish-gray coating at base, Nat-s.); tip and edges red; right side of throat and neck most affected.

For Hunterian (hard) chancre, secondary symptoms rarely follow if given in proper dose; great swelling of inguinal glands, no disposition to suppurate.

MERCURIUS SOLUBILIS

Hahnemann's Soluble Mercury   *Black Oxide*

Nervous affections after suppressed discharges especially in psoric patients (Asaf.).

Glandular and scrofulous affections of children.

Otorrhea: Bloody, offensive discharge, with stabbing, tearing pain; < right side, at night and lying on affected side.

Furuncles and boils in external meatus (Pic-ac.).

Polypi and fungus excrescences in external meatus (Teucr., Thuj.).

Acrid nasal secretion, having odor of old cheese; nostrils, red, raw, ulcerated.

Epistaxis: When coughing; *at night during sleep*; hangs in *a dark clotted string* from the nose, like an icicle.

Gonorrhea: With phimosis or chancroids; *green discharge, < at night;* urging to urinate; intolerable burning in forepart of urethra when passing last few drops; prepuce hot, swollen, edematous and sensitive to touch; of a torpid character, with threatening or suppurating bubo.

Chancre: Primary; regular indurated Hunterian, with lardaceous base; with cheesy bottom and inverted red edges; with phimosis or paraphimosis; deep, round, penetrating, eating through fraenum and prepuce; bleeding, painful; yellowish, fetid discharge.

Hahnemann's remedy for syphilis and diseases of the genito-urinary tract. Is rarely indicated if the tongue is dry.

Diseases of the skin; intolerable biting, itching, over body, as from insect bites, < in evening and from warmth of bed; becomes pleasant on scratching.

Weakness and weariness of limbs; sore, bruised.

MERCURIUS SULPHURICUS

Sulphate of Mercury $HgSO_4$

Hydrothorax, if occurring from heart or liver diseases; dyspnea, has to sit, cannot lie down. Extremities swollen; stool loose, watery, causing severe burning and soreness; burning in chest.

"When it acts well it produces a profuse, watery diarrhea with great relief to the patient; it is as important as Arsenicum in hydrothorax." – Lippe.

Relationship

Compare: Ars., Cinnb., Dig., Sulph.

MEZEREUM

Daphne Mezereum   *Thymelaceae*

For light-haired, irresolute persons of a phlegmatic temperament.

Eczema and itching eruptions *after vaccination*.

Hypochondriacal and despondent; indifferent to everything and every one; angry at trifles and perfectly harmless things, but is soon sorry for it.

Toothache: In carious teeth (Kreos.); feel elongated, dull pain when biting on them and when touched with tongue, < at night; > with mouth open and drawing in air; roots decay (reverse of Merc.).

Headache, violent after slight vexation; painful on the slightest touch; right-sided.

The head is covered with **thick, leather-like crust,** under which thick and white pus collects here and there; hair is glued and matted together; pus after a time is ichorous, becomes offensive and breeds vermin.

Ulcers with thick, yellowish-white scabs, under which thick, yellow pus collects.

Vesicles appear around the ulcers, itch violently, burn like fire (Hep.); shining, fiery-red areola around.

Linen or charpie sticks to the ulcers, they bleed when it is torn away.

Eczema: Intolerable itching, < in bed and from touch; copious, serous exudation.

Neuralgic burning pains after zona.

Bones, especially long bones, inflamed, swollen; nightly pains going from above downwards; after abuse of Merc., after venereal diseases; caries, exostosis, tumors soften from within out.

Pain in periosteum of long bones < at night in bed, least touch, in damp weather (Merc., Phyt.).

Child scratches face continuously, which is covered with blood; eruptions moist; itching worse at night; inflammatory redness of face.

Relationship

Compare: Caust., Guaj., Phyt., Rhus-t.

Aggravation

Cold air; cold washing; at night; touch or motion; bad effects of mercury or alcohol.

Epidemics occurring in January and February often call for Mezereum.

MILLEFOLIUM

Yarrow *Compositae*

Ailments: From over-lifting, over-exertion, or a fall.

Vertigo: When moving slowly, but not when taking violent exercise.

Hemorrhages: Painless, without fever; bright red, fluid blood (Acon., Ip., Sab.); from lungs, bronchi, larynx, mouth, nose, stomach, bladder, rectum, uterus; of mechanical origin (Arn.); of wounds (Ham.).

Wounds which bleed profusely, *especially after a fall* (Arn., Ham.).

Hemoptysis: After injury; in incipient phthisis; in hemorrhoidal patients; from a ruptured blood vessel.

Painless drainage, from nose, lungs, uterus; after labor or abortion; after great exertion; after miscarriage. Preventive in post-partum hemorrhage.

Menses: Early, *profuse, protracted*; suppressed, with colic pain in abdomen.

Leucorrhea of children from atony (Calc.).

Cough: With raising of bright blood; in suppressed menses or hemorrhoids; with oppression and palpitation; after a fall from a height (Arn.); after violent exertion; with blood, daily at 4 p.m. (Lyc.).

Relationship

Compare: Erech. in epistaxis and hemoptysis, blood bright red.

Follows well: After, Acon. and Arn. in hemorrhages.

MUREX PURPUREA

A Mollusc   *Muricidae*

Persons of a melancholy temperament.

For the sufferings during climacteric (Lach., Sep., Sulph.). Great depression of spirits.

Sinking, all gone sensation, in stomach (Sep.).

Least contact of parts causes violent sexual excitement (excessive sexual irritation driving to self abuse, Orig., Zinc.).

Violent excitement in sexual organs, and excessive desire for an embrace (reverse of, Sep.).

Sore pain in uterus; a distinct sensation of a womb (Helon., Lyss.)

Bearing down sensation, as if internal organs would be pushed out, must sit down and cross limbs to > pressure (but no sexual desire, Sep.).

Menses: Irregular, early, profuse, protracted, large clots.

Leucorrhea: < mental depression, happier when leucorrhea is worse.

Relationship

Compare: Lil-t., Plat., in nymphomania; Sep. in bearing down sensation, but has no sexual erethism.

MURIATICUM ACIDUM

Hydrochloric Acid   *HCl*

Adapted to persons with black hair, dark eyes, dark complexion.

Irritable, peevish, disposed to anger and chagrin (Nux-v.); restlessness and vertigo.

Diseases of an asthenic type, with moaning, unconsciousness, fretfulness.

MURIATICUM ACIDUM

Ulceration with fungus-like growths and pseudo-like membranous deposits of intestinal tract.

Great debility; as soon as he sits down his eyes close; **lower jaw hangs down; slides down in bed.**

Mouth and anus are chiefly affected; the tongue and sphincter ani are paralyzed.

Malignant affections of mouth; studded with ulcers, deep, perforating; having a black or dark base; offensive, foul breath; intense prostration; diphtheria, scarlatina, cancer.

Cannot bear the thought or sight of meat (Nit-ac.).

If the anus be very sensitive either with or without hemorrhoids; anus sore during menses.

Hemorrhoids: *Swollen, blue,* **sensitive and painful to touch;** appear *suddenly in children;* too sore to bear least touch, even the sheet is uncomfortable. *Prolapse while urinating.*

Diarrhea: Stool involuntary *while urinating; on passing wind* (Aloe); cannot urinate *without having the bowels move at the same time.*

Urine passes slowly; bladder weak, must wait a long time; has to press so that anus protrudes.

Cannot bear least touch, not even of sheet on genitals (Murx.).

Typhoid or typhus; deep stupid sleep; unconscious while awake; loud moaning or muttering; tongue coated at edges, *shrunken, dry, leather-like, paralyzed;* involuntary fetid stools *while passing urine; sliding down in bed;* pulse intermits every third beat.

Palpitation of heart is felt in the face.

Freckles; eczema solaris.

Relationship

Follows well: After, Bry., Merc., Rhus-t.

Cures the muscular weakness following excessive use of opium and tobacco.

NAJA TRIPUDIANS

Cobra Virus   *Elapidae*

Suicidal insanity, broods constantly over imaginary troubles (Aur.).

Simple hypertrophy of heart.

For restoring a heart damaged by acute inflammation, or from relief of sufferings of chronic hypertrophy and valvular lesions.

Irritating, dry, sympathetic cough in the acute stage of rheumatic carditis, or chronic organic lesions (Spong.).

Threatened paralysis of heart, post-diphtheritic.

Pulse irregular in force, but regular in rhythm.

Inability to speak with choking, nervous, chronic palpitation, especially after public speaking; pain < by carriage riding or lying on side.

Severe stitching pain in region of heart.

Relationship

Compare: Ars., Cact., Crot-h., Lach., Mygal., Spig.

NATRIUM CARBONICUM

Carbonate of Soda $Na_2CO_3.10H_2O$

Constitutions with aversion to open air and dislike to exercise, mental or physical; imbecility.

Great debility; **caused by heat of summer** (Ant-c.); exhaustion *from least effort,* mental or physical; ready to drop after a walk; **chronic effects of sunstroke.**

Chronic effects of sunstroke; now, with return of hot weather, suffers from headaches.

Emaciation with pale face and blue rings around the eyes, dilated pupils; dark urine; anemic; milky, watery skin and great debility.

Inability to think or to perform any mental labor; causes headache; feels stupefied if he tries to exert himself; comprehension slow, difficult.

Intolerable melancholy and apprehension; is wholly occupied with sad thoughts.

Attacks of anxiety and restlessness during a thunderstorm (Phos.); < from music (Sab.).

Headache: From slightest mental exertion; from *sun* or *working under gaslight* (Glon., Lach.); with tension in nape or occiput before menses; head feels too large, as if it would burst.

Face pale, with blue rings around the eyes; eyelids swollen; catarrh; mucus in throat and posterior nares; constantly hawking to clear the throat; dropping into the throat from posterior nares.

Catarrh: Extends to posterior nares and throat; hawking much thick mucus from throat; profuse discharge during day, stopped at night (Nux-v.).

Thick, yellow, green offensive, musty, hard discharge from nose; often ceasing after a meal.

Aversion to milk; diarrhoea from it.

Bearing down as if everything would come out (Agar., Lil-t., Murx., Sep.); heaviness, < sitting, > by moving.

Discharge of mucus from vagina after an embrace, causing sterility.

Easy dislocation and spraining of ankle (Led.); so weak that it gives way; foot bends under (Carb-an., Nat-m.).

Relationship

Compare: Nat-s., for yeast-like vomiting; Calc., Sep.

Follows well: After, Sep. in bearing down.

Aggravation

From music; *in the sun;* excessive summer heat; *mental exertion;* a thunderstorm.

NATRIUM MURIATICUM

Common Salt *NaCl*

For the anemic and cathectic; whether *form loss of vital fluids* – profuse menses, seminal losses – or mental affections.

NATRIUM MURIATICUM

Great emaciation; losing flesh while living well (Abrot., Iod.); throat and neck of children emaciate rapidly during summer complaint (Sanic.).

Great liability to take cold (Calc., Kali-c.).

Irritability: Child cross when spoken to; crying from slightest cause; gets into a passion about trifles, especially when consoled with.

Awkward, hasty, drops things from nervous weakness (Apis, Bov.).

Marked disposition to weep; sad weeping mood, without cause (Puls.), but consolation from other < her troubles.

Headache: Anemic, of school girls (Calc-p.); *from sunrise to sunset;* left-sided clavus; as if bursting; with red face, nausea and vomiting before, during and after menses; as though a thousand little hammers were knocking in the brain during fever; > by perspiration.

Headache; *beginning with blindness* (Iris, Kali-bi.); with zig-zag dazzling, like lightning in eyes, ushering in a throbbing headache; from eye strain.

Lachrymation; tears stream down the face whenever he coughs (Euphr.).

Hay fever: Squirming sensation in the nostril, as of a small worm; brought on by exposure to hot sun or intense summer heat.

Sensation as of a hair on the tongue (Sil.).

Tongue: **Mapped,** *with red insular patches;* like ringworm on sides (Ars., Lach., Merc., Nit-ac., Tarax.); heavy, difficult speech, *children slow in learning to walk.*

Constipation: Sensation of contraction of anus; torn, bleeding, smarting afterwards; stool dry, hard, difficult, crumbling (Am-c., Mag-m.); stitches in rectum (Nit-ac.); involuntary, knows not whether flatus or feces escape (Aloe, Iod., Mur-ac., Olnd., Podo.).

Urine: Involuntary when walking, coughing, laughing (Caust., Puls., Squil.); has to wait a long while for urine to pass, *if others are present* (Hep., Mur-ac.); cutting in urethra *after* (Sars.).

Seminal emission: Soon after coition, with increased desire; weakness of organs with retarded emission during an embrace; impotence, spinal irritation, paralysis, after sexual excesses.

Pressing, pushing towards genitals every morning; must sit down to prevent prolapsus (Lil-t., Murx., Sep.).

Fluttering of the heart; with a weak faint feeling < lying down (Lach.).

The heart's pulsations shake the body (Spig.).

The hair falls out when touched, in nursing women (Sep.); face oily, shiny, as if greased (Plb., Thuj.).

For the bad effects: Of anger (caused by offence); acid food, bread, quinine, excessive use of salts, of cauterization of all kinds with the silver nitrate; of grief, fright, vexation, mortification or reserved displeasure (Staph.)

Hangnails: Skin around the nails dry and cracked (Graph., Petr.); herpes about anus and on borders of hair at nape of neck (in bend of knees, Hep., Graph.).

Warts on palms of hands (sore to touch, Nat-c.).

Dreams: *Of robbers* in the house, and on waking will not believe to the contrary until search is made (Psor.); of burning thirst.

Fever blisters, *like pearls* about the lips; lips dry, sore and cracked, ulcerated (Nit-ac.).

Painful contractions of the hamstrings (Am-m., Caust., Guaj.).

Craving for salt (Calc., Caust.); great aversion to bread.

Eczema; raw, red, inflamed, especially in edges of hair; < from eating too much salt, at sea shore, or from ocean voyage.

Urticaria, acute or chronic; over whole body, especially after violent exercise (Apis, Calc., Hep., Sanic., Urt-u.).

Intermittent: *Paroxysm at* 10 *or* 11 a.m.; old, chronic, badly treated cases, especially after suppression by quinine; headache, with unconsciousness during chill and heat; sweat > pains.

Relationship

Complementary: To, Apis; acts well before and after it.

Natrium mur. is the chronic of Ignatia, which is its vegetable analogue.

Is followed by Sepia and Thuja.

Cannot often be repeated in chronic cases without an intercurrent, called for by the symptoms.

Should never be given during fever paroxysm.

NATRIUM MURIATICUM—NATRIUM SULPHURICUM

If vertigo and headache be very persistent, or prostration be prolonged after Natrium, Nux will relieve.

Aggravation

At 10 *or* 11 a.m.; at the seashore or from sea air; heat of sun or stove; mental exertion, talking, writing, reading; lying down.

Amelioration

In the open air (Apis, Puls.); cold bathing; *going, without regular meals;* lying on right side (on painful side, Bry., Ign., Puls.).

NATRUM SULPHURICUM

Sodium Sulphate $NaOSO_3 \cdot 10Aq$

Ailments which are < by, or which depend upon, *dampness of weather, damp houses or cellars* (Aran.).

Patient feels every change from dry to wet; cannot tolerate sea air, nor eat plants that thrive near water; a constitution in which the gonorrheal poison is most pernicious; recovers slowly from every sickness.

Every spring, skin affections reappear (Psor.).

Inability to think (Nat-c.).

Sad, gloomy, irritable; worse in morning; dislikes to speak or be spoken to (Iod., Sil.).

Depressed; *lively music makes her sad;* satiety of life; must use great self-control to prevent shooting himself.

NATRIUM SULPHURICUM

Mental traumatism; mental effects from injuries to head; chronic brain effects of blows, falls.

Granular lids: *Like small blisters* (Thuja); green pus and terrible photophobia; gonorrheal or sycotic.

Nosebleed during menses (instead of menses, Bry., Puls.).

Toothache > by cold water, cool air (Coff., Puls.).

Dirty, greenish-gray or brown coating on tongue.

Diarrhea: Sudden, urging, gushing, much flatus; *on first rising and standing on the feet;* after a spell of wet weather; living or working in basements.

Gonorrhea: *Greenish-yellow, painless,* thick discharge (Puls.); chronic or suppressed (thick, green Kali-i.).

Dyspnea: Desire to take a deep breath during damp, cloudy weather.

Humid asthma in children; *with every change to wet weather;* with every fresh cold; always worse in damp, rainy weather; sputa green, greenish, copious (greenish-gray, Cop.).

Sycotic pneumonia: *Lower lobe of left lung;* great soreness of chest, during cough, has to sit up in bed and hold the chest with both hands (Nicc.; right lung, Bry.).

Spinal meningitis: Violent, *crushing gnawing pains at base of brain;* head drawn back; spasms with mental irritability and delirium; violent congestion of blood to head; delirium; opisthotonos.

Relationship

Compare: Nat-m. and Sulph., which are very similar; Thuj. and Merc. in syphilis and sycosis occurring in hydrogenoid constitutions.

Aggravation

Damp basements or dwellings; damp weather (Aran., Ars-i., Dulc.); rest; lying.

Amelioration

Dry weather; pressure, sitting up (cough); changing position (but > in wet weather, Caust.); open air.

Must change position frequently, but it is painful and gives little relief (Caust.).

NITRICUM ACIDUM

Nitric Acid HNO_3

Especially suited to thin persons of rigid fibre, dark complexions, black hair and eyes—the brunette rather than the blonde—nervous temperament.

Persons suffering with chronic diseases who take cold easily; are easily disposed to diarrhea; rarely to those who suffer with constipation.

Old people with great weakness and diarrhea.

Excessive *physical* irritability.

Pains: **Sticking, pricking as from splinters;** suddenly appearing and disappearing; on change of

NITRICUM ACIDUM

temperature or weather; during sleep; gnawing here and there as from ulcers forming.

Sensation: Of a band around head, around the bones (Carb-ac., Sulph.); *of a splinter* in affected parts, ulcers, piles, throat, ingrowing toe nail < on slightest contact.

Ailments: Which depend on some virulent poison; from mercury, syphilis, scrofula, in broken-down cachectic constitutions.

After continued loss of sleep, long-lasting anxiety, over-exertion of mind and body from nursing the sick (Cocc.); anguish from the loss of his dearest friend; indifference; tired of life; sadness before menses.

Great anxiety about his disease; constantly thinking about his past troubles; morbid fear of cholera (Ars.); depressed and anxious in the evening.

Irritable, headstrong; hateful and vindictive; inveterate, ill-willed, unmoved by apologies.

Hardness of hearing > by riding in carriage or train (Graph.).

Very sensitive to rattle of wagons over paved streets; headache from pressure of hat (Calc-p., Carb-v., Nat-m.).

Ozena: Green casts from the nose every morning.

Diarrhea: Great straining but little passes, as if feces remained and cannot be expelled (Alum.); pain as if rectum or anus were torn or fissured (Nat-m.); violent cutting pains *after stool,* lasting for hours (Rat., Sulph.; during and after, Merc.).

Fissures in rectum; tearing, spasmodic pains during stools; lancinating, even after soft stools (Alumn., Nat-m., Rat.).

Urine: *Scanty, dark-brown,* **strong-smelling,** "like horse's urine"; *cold when it passes;* turbid, looks like remains of a cider barrel.

Ulcers: Easily bleeding; in corners of mouth (Nat-m.); *splinter-like pains,* especially on contact (Hep.); zig-zag, irregular edges; base looks like raw flesh; exuberant granulations; after mercury or syphilis or both, engrafted on a scrofulous base.

Discharges: Thin, offensive, acrid; of a brown or dirty yellowish-green color, rarely laudable pus.

Hemorrhage: From bowels in typhoid or typhus (Crot-h., Mur-ac.); after miscarriage or post-partum; from over-exertion of body; bright, profuse, or dark.

Cracking: In ears, on masticating; of the joints, on motion (Cocc., Graph.).

Warts, condylomata; sycotic or syphilitic; large, jagged, pedunculated; bleeding readily on washing; moist, oozing; sticking pain (Staph., Thuj.).

Affects especially the mucus outlets of the body where skin and mucous membrane join; mouth, nose, rectum, anus, urethra, vagina (Mur-ac.).

Relationship

Complementary: Ars. and Calad.

Inimical: To, Lachesis.

Resembles: Ars. in morbid fear of cholera.

Often difficult to distinguish from Merc.; but is adapted to black-haired people, while Merc. is more useful in light-haired persons.

Relieves ailments resulting from abuse of mercury, especially if there be erethism; bad effects of repeated doses of Digitalis.

Follows well: Calc., Hep., Merc., Nat-c., Puls. or Thuj.; but is most effective after Kali-c.

Aggravation

Evening and at night; after midnight; contact; change of temperature or weather; during sweat; on walking; while walking.

Amelioration

While riding in a carriage (reverse of Cocc.).

NUX MOSCHATA

Nutmeg　　　　　　　　　　　　　*Myristicaceae*

Adapted especially to women and children of a nervous hysterical temperament (Ign.); to people with a *dry skin, who rarely perspire;* complaints of pregnancy.

Weakness of old age; dyspepsia of old people.

Oversensitive: To light; of hearing; of smell; to touch.

All the ailments are accompanied by **drowsiness and sleepiness** (Ant-t., Op.) *or an inclination to faint* even from slight pain (Hep.); **complaints cause sleepiness.**

Stupor and insensibility; unconquerable sleep.

Absence of mind; cannot think; indifference to everything.

Weakness or loss of memory (Anac., Lac-c., Lyc.).

Vanishing of thoughts while reading, talking or writing; uses wrong words; does not recognize well-known streets (Cann-i., Lach.).

Changeable humor; one moment laughing, the next crying (Croc., Ign.); "sudden change from grave to gay, from lively to serene" (Plat.).

Dryness of eyes; too dry to close the lids.

Great dryness of the mouth (Apis, Lach.); *tongue so dry it adheres to roof of mouth;* saliva seemed like cotton; throat dry, stiffened, no thirst (Puls.).

Sensation of great dryness without real thirst and without actual dryness of the tongue.

Great soreness of all the parts upon which one lies (Bapt., Pyrog.); tendency to bedsores.

Eating a little too much causes headache; painfulness and distress in stomach *while eating* or immediately after (Kali-bi.).

Abdomen enormously distended after every meal.

Diarrhea: In summer, from *cold drinks;* epidemic in autumn, white stools (Colch.); from boiled milk; during dentition; during pregnancy; with sleepiness and fainting; in autumn, epidemic, white, fetid (Colch.).

At every menstrual nisus, mouth, throat and tongue become intolerably dry, especially when sleeping.

Leucorrhea in place of menses (Cocc.); patient awakened with dry tongue (Lach.); physometra (Lac-c., Lyc.).

Pain, nausea and vomiting during pregnancy; from wearing pessaries.

Sudden hoarseness, < from walking against the wind (Euphr., Hep.).

Cough caused by: Getting warm in bed; being overheated; during pregnancy (Con.); bathing, standing in water; living in cold, damp places (Nat-s.); loose after eating, dry after drinking.

Sleep: Irresistibly drowsy; sleepy, muddled, as if intoxicated; coma, lies silent, immovable; eyes constantly closed (with stertorous breathing, Op.).

Rheumatic affections; from getting feet wet; from exposure to drafts of air while heated (Acon., Bry.); < in cold, wet weather, or cold wet clothes (Rhus-t.); of left shoulder (Ferr.).

Backache, while riding in a carriage.

Fatigue, must lie down after the least exertion.

Relationship

Nux moschata antidotes mercurial inhalation, lead colic, oil of turpentine, spirituous liquors, and especially the effects of bad beer.

Aggravation

Cold, wet windy weather (Rhod.); weather changes; cold food, water and cold washing; carriage driving (Cocc.); lying on painful side (on painless side, Puls.).

Amelioration

In dry, warm weather; warm room; wrapping up warmly.

NUX VOMICA

Poison Nut   *Loganiaceae*

Adapted to thin, irritable, careful, zealous persons with dark hair and bilious or sanguine temperament. Disposed to be *quarrelsome, spiteful, malicious;* nervous and melancholic.

Debauchers of a *thin, irritable, nervous disposition,* prone to indigestion and hemorrhoids (persons with light hair, blue eyes, Lob.).

"Nux is chiefly successful with persons of an ardent character; of an irritable, impatient temperament, disposed to anger, spite or deception."—Hahnemann.

Anxiety with irritability and inclination to commit suicide, but is afraid to die.

Hypochondriac: Literary, studious persons, who are too much at home, suffer from want of exercise, with gastric, abdominal complaints and costiveness; especially in drunkards.

Oversensitive: *To external impressions; to noise, odors, light or music* (Nux-m.); *trifling ailments are unbearable* (Cham.); every harmless word offends (Ign.).

Persons who are very particular, careful, but inclined to become easily excited or angered; irascible and tenacious.

Bad effects of: Coffee, tobacco, alcoholic stimulants; highly spiced or seasoned food; over-eating (Ant-c.); long-continued mental over-exertion; sedentary habits; loss of sleep (Cocc., Colch., Nit-ac.); aromatic or patent

NUX VOMICA

medicine; sitting on cold stones, especially in warm weather.

One of the best remedies with which to commence treatment of cases that have been drugged by mixtures, bitters, vegetable pills, nostrums or quack remedies, especially aromatic or "hot medicines," *but only if symptoms correspond.*

Convulsions, *with consciousness* (Strych.); < anger, *emotion, touch, moving.*

Pains are tingling, sticking, hard, aching, worse from motion and contact.

Tendency to faint (Nux-m., Sulph.); from odors; in morning; after eating; after every labor pain.

Cannot keep from falling asleep in the evening while sitting or reading hours before bedtime, and awakes at 3 or 4 a.m.; falls into a dreamy sleep at daybreak from which he is hard to arouse, and then feels tired and weak (reverse of, Puls.).

Catarrh: Snuffles of infants (Am-c., Samb.); coryza, dry at night, fluent by day; < in warm room, > in cold air; from sitting in cold places, on stone steps.

Eructations: Sour, bitter; nausea and vomiting every morning with depression of spirits; after eating.

Nausea: Constant; after eating; in morning; from smoking; and feels "If I could only vomit I would be so much better."

Stomach: Pressure an hour or two after eating as from a stone (immediately after, Kali-bi., Nux-m.); pyrosis, tightness, must loosen clothing; cannot use the mind for two or three hours after a meal; sleepy after dinner; from anxiety, worry, brandy, coffee, drugs, night watching, high living, etc.

Constipation; with frequent unsuccessful desire, passing small quantities of feces (in upper abdomen, Ign., Verat.); sensation as if not finished.

Frequent desire for stool; anxious, ineffectual, > for a time after stool; in morning after rising; after mental exertion (inactive, no desire, Bry., Sulph.).

Alternate constipation and diarrhea (Sulph., Verat.), in persons who have taken purgatives all their lives.

Menses: Too early, profuse, lasts too long; or keeping on several days longer, with complaints at onset and remaining after; every two weeks; irregular, never at right time; stopping and starting again (Sulph.); during and after, < of old symptoms.

Labor pains: *Violent*, spasmodic; cause urging to *stool or to urinate*; < in back; prefers a warm room.

Strangulated hernia, especially umbilical.

Backache: Must sit up or turn over in bed; lumbago; from sexual weakness, from masturbation.

Repugnance to cold or to cold air; chilly, on least movement; from being uncovered; **must be covered in every stage of fever**—chill, heat or sweat.

Fever: Great heat, whole body burning hot (Acon.), face red and hot (Bell.), yet patient *cannot move or uncover without being chilly.*

Relationship

Complementary: Sulphur in early all diseases.

Inimical: To, Zinc.; must not be used before or after.

Follows well: After, Ars., Ip., Phos., Sep., Sulph.

Is followed well: By, Bry., Puls., Sulph.

Nux should be given on retiring or, what is better, several hours before going to bed; it acts best during repose of mind and body.

Aggravation

Morning; waking at 4 a.m.; *mental exertion;* after eating or over-eating; touch, noise, anger, spices, narcotics, dry weather; in cold air.

Amelioration

In evening, while at rest; lying down, and in damp wet weather (Caust.).

OPIUM

Poppy *Papaveraceae*

Especially adapted to children and old people; diseases of first and second childhood (Bar-c., Mill.), persons with light hair, lax muscles, and want of bodily irritability.

Want of susceptibility to remedies; lack of vital reaction, the well chosen remedy makes no impression (Carb-v., Laur., Valer.).

Ailments: With insensibility and partial or complete paralysis; that originate *from fright*, bad effects of, the fear still remaining (Acon., Hyos.); from charcoal vapors; from inhaling gas; of drunkards.

All complaints: With great sopor; painless, complains of nothing; wants nothing.

Spasms: Of children, from approach of strangers; from nursing after fright of mother (Hyos.; after anger of mother, Cham., Nux-v.); from crying; eyes half open and upturned.

Screaming before or during a spasm (Apis, Hell.). Deep stertorous respiration both on inhalation and exhalation.

Delirium: Constantly talking; eyes wide open, face red, puffed; or unconscious, eyes glassy, half-closed, face pale, deep coma preceded by stupor.

Thinks she is not at home (Bry.); this is continually in her mind.

Picking of bed clothes during sleep (while awake, Bell., Hyos.).

Delirium tremens: In old emaciated persons; bloated face, stupor, eyes burning, hot dry; with loud snoring.

Sleep: Heavy, stupid; **with stertorous breathing,** *red face, eyes half closed,* blood-shot; *skin covered with hot sweat;* after convulsions.

Sleepy, but cannot sleep (Bell., Cham.), sleeplessness with acuteness of hearing, clock striking and cocks crowing at a great distance keep her awake.

Loss of breath on falling asleep (Grind., Lach.).

Bed feels so hot she cannot lie on it (bed feels hard, Arn., Bry., Pyrog.); moves often in search of a cool place; must be uncovered.

Digestive organs inactive; peristaltic motion reversed or paralyzed; bowels seem closed.

Constipation: Of children; of corpulent, good-natured women (Graph.); from inaction or paresis, no desire; from lead poisoning; stool hard, round, black balls (Chel., Plb., Thuj.); feces protrude and recede (Sil., Thuj.).

Stool: Involuntary, especially after fright (Gels.); *black and offensive; from paralysis of sphincter.*

Urine: Retained, with bladder full; retention, postpartum or from excessive use of tobacco; in nursing children, after passion of nurse; in fever or acute illness; paralysis of bladder or sphincter.

(In Stramonium we have suppression; while in Opium the secretion in not diminished, the bladder is full but fullness is unrecognized.)

Opium renders the intestines so sluggish that the most active purgatives lose their power. – Hering.

Persistent diarrhea in those treated with large doses of the drug.—Lippe.

Sudden retrocession of acute exanthema results in paralysis of brain or convulsions (Zinc.).

Marasmus; child with wrinkled skin, looks like a little dried up old man (Abrot.).

Relationship

Antidotes, for poisonous doses; strong coffee, Nux-v., Kali-perm. and constant motion.

When symptoms correspond, the potencies may antidote bad effects of Opium drugging.

Compare: Apis, Bell., Hyos., Stram., and Zinc.

Aggravation

During and after sleep (Apis, Lach.); while perspiring; from warmth; stimulants.

Amelioration

From cold; constant walking.

PETROLEUM

Coal or Rock Oil *Anthracite*

Adapted to persons with light hair and skin; irritable, quarrelsome disposition (Nux-v.); easily offended at trifles (Ign., Med.); vexed at everything.

Ailments: From riding in a carriage, railroad car, or in a ship (Cocc., Sanic.).

Ailments which are worse before and during a thunderstorm (Nat-c., Phos., Psor.).

Symptoms appear and disappear rapidly (Bell., Mag-p.; reverse of, Plat., Stann.).

During sleep or delirium: Imagines that one leg is

double; *that another person lies alongside of him in same bed; that there are two babies in the bed* (Valer.).

Vertigo on rising (Bry.); *in occiput;* as if intoxicated; *like sea sickness* (Cocc.).

Headache: *In occiput, which is as heavy as lead;* pressing, pulsating pain; as if everything in the head were alive; numb, bruised; as if made of wood.

Gastralgia: Of pregnancy; with pressing, drawing pains; *whenever stomach is empty; relieved by constant eating* (All-c., Anac., Chel.).

Diarrhea: Yellow, watery, *gushing;* after cabbage, sour krout; during pregnancy, stormy weather; *always in the daytime.*

Painful sensitiveness of skin of whole body; all clothing is painful; slight injury suppurates (Hep.).

Skin of hands rough, cracked; *tips of fingers* rough, cracked, fissured, *every winter;* tenderness of the feet, which are bathed in foul-smelling sweat (Graph., Sanic., Sil.).

Herpes: Of genital organs extending to perineum and thighs; itching, redness; skin cracked, rough, bleeding; dry or moist.

Heat and burning of soles of feet and palms of hands (Sang., Sulph.).

Sweat and moisture of external genitals, both sexes.

Painful, itching chilblains and chapped hands < in cold weather; decubitus.

Sensation of coldness about the heart (Carb-an., Kali-m., Nat-m.).

Relationship

One of our best antidotes for lead poisoning.

The skin symptoms are worse in winter, better in summer (Alum.); if suppressed, causes diarrhea.

Aggravation

Carriage riding (Cocc., Sanic.); during a thunderstorm; *in winter* (Alum.).

PETROSELINUM

Parsley   *Umbelliferae*

Intermittent fever: Complicating traumatic or chronic urethritis or stricture; with abdominal affections and perverted or defective assimilation.

Thirsty and hungry yet as soon as they begin to eat or drink they lose all desire (reverse of Calc.).

Sudden urging to urinate (Canth.).

Child suddenly seized with desire to urinate; if cannot be gratified at once *jumps up and down with pain.*

Burning, tingling *from perineum throughout whole urethra.*

Frequent voluptuous tickling in fossa navicularis.

Gonorrhea: Sudden irresistible desire to urinate; *intense biting, itching,* deep in urethra, must rub it with some rough article in urethra for >; pain at root of penis or neck of bladder. Gleet.

Relationship

Compare: Cann-i., Canth., Merc. in sudden urging to urinate.

PHOSPHORICUM ACIDUM

Glacial Phosphoric Acid HPO_3

Best suited to persons of originally strong constitutions, who have become debilitated **by loss of vital fluids,** sexual excesses (Chin.); violent acute diseases; chagrin, or a long succession of moral emotions, as grief, care, disappointed affection.

Ailments: From care, chagrin, grief, sorrow, home sickness (Ign.); sleepy, disposed to weep; night-sweats towards morning.

Pale, sickly complexion, eyes sunken and surrounded by blue margins (Puls.).

Is listless, apathetic: *Indifferent to the affairs of life; prostrated and stupefied with grief,* to those things that used to be of most interest, especially if there be debility and emaciation.

Delirium: Muttering, unintelligible; lies in a stupor, or a stupid sleep, unconscious of all that is going on around him; when aroused is fully conscious, answers slowly and correctly and relapses into stupor.

In children and young people who grow too rapidly (Calc., Calc-p.); pains in back and limbs as if beaten.

Headache: *Crushing weight on vertex,* from long-lasting grief or exhausted nerves; in occiput and nape; usually from behind forward, < by least motion, noise, especially music, > lying (Bry., Gels., Sil.).

Headache of school girls from eye strain or overuse of eyes (Calc-p., Nat-m.); of students who are growing too fast.

Patient trembles, legs weak, stumbles easily or makes mis-steps; weak and indifferent to the affairs of life.

Interstitial inflammation of bones, scrofulous, sycotic, syphilitic, mercurial; periosteum inflamed, pains burning, tearing, as if scraped with a knife (Rhus-t.); caries, rachitis, but not necrosis; growing pains.

Boring, drawing, digging pains in nerves of extremities, necrosis in stump after amputations (All-c).

Diarrhea: *Painless; not debilitating; white* or yellow, watery; from acids, involuntary, with the flatus (Aloe, Nat-m.); cholereic, from fear.

Urine: Looks like milk mixed with jelly-like, bloody pieces; decomposes rapidly; *profuse urination at night of clear, watery urine,* which forms a white cloud at once (phosphates in excess, nerve waste).

Onanism; when patient is greatly distressed by the capability of the act (compare Dios., Staph.).

Emission: *Frequent, profuse, debilitating;* after coitus; most desire, after; several in one night; *abashed, sad, despair of cure* (with irresistible tendency to masturbate, Ust.).

Chest: Weak from talking or coughing (Stann.); in phthisis; nervous from loss of vital fluids, too rapid growth, depressing mental emotions.

Cerebral typhoid or typhus: **Complete apathy and stupor;** takes no notice, "lies like a log," utterly regardless of surrounding; intestinal hemorrhage, blood dark.

Relationship

Compare: Phos., Puls., Pic-ac., Sil.; Mur-ac. in typhoid; Nit-s-d. in apathetic stupor and delirium.

Ph-ac. acts well before or after Chin. in colliquative sweats, diarrhea, debility; after Nux-v. in fainting after a meal.

Aggravation

From mental affections; loss of vital fluids; especially seminal; self abuse; sexual excesses; talking causes weakness in chest (Stann.).

PHOSPHORUS

Phosphorus *The Element*

Adapted to *tall slender persons* of sanguine temperament, fair skin, *delicate eyelashes, fine blond, or red hair,* quick perceptions, and very sensitive nature.

Young people who grow too rapidly, are inclined to stoop (to walk stooped, Sulph.); who are chlorotic or anemia; old people, with morning diarrhea.

PHOSPHORUS

Nervous, weak; desires to be magnetised (Sil.).

Oversensitiveness of all the senses to external impressions, light, noise, odors, touch.

Restless, fidgety; moves continually, cannot sit or stand still a moment (restless, fidgety feet, Zinc.).

Burning: *In spots* along the spine; *between the scapulae* (as of a piece of ice, Lachn.); or intense heat running up the back; of palms of hands (Lach.); in chest and lungs; of every organ or tissue of the body (Ars., Sulph.); generally in diseases of nervous system.

Hemorrhage diathesis; small wounds bleed profusely (Kreos., Lach.); from every mucous outlet.

Great weakness and prostration; with nervous debility and trembling; of whole body; weakness and weariness from loss of vital fluids (Chin., Ph-ac.).

Pain: Acute especially in the chest, < from pressure, even slight, *in intercostal spaces, and lying on left side;* excited by slightest chill; open air intolerable.

A weak, empty, all-gone sensation in head, chest, stomach and *entire abdomen.*

Apathetic; unwilling to talk; answers slowly; moves sluggishly (Ph-ac.).

Weary of life, full of gloomy forebodings.

Dandruff, falls out in clouds (Lyc.); hair falls out in bunches, baldness of single spots.

Eyes: Hollow, surrounded *by blue rings;* lids, puffy, swollen, edematous (upper lids, Kali-c.; lower, Apis).

Longs for: Cold food and drink; juicy refreshing things; ice cream > gastric pains.

As soon as water becomes warm in stomach it is thrown up.

Rugurgitation of ingesta, in mouthfuls (Alum.).

Nausea from placing hands in warm water; sneezing and coryza from putting hands in water (Lac-d.).

Constipation: Feces slender, long, dry, tough and hard (Staph.); voided with great straining and difficulty (Caust.).

Diarrhea: As soon as anything *enters the rectum;* profuse, pouring away as from a hydrant; watery, with sago-like particles; *sensation,* **as if the anus remained open** (Apis); involuntary during cholera time (which precedes cholera, Ph-ac.); morning, of old people.

Hemorrhage: Frequent and profuse, pouring out freely and then ceasing for a time; metrorrhagia, in cancer, hemoptysis vicarious, from nose, stomach, anus, urethra, in amenorrhea.

Heaviness of chest, as if a weight were lying on it.

During pregnancy; unable to drink water; slight of it causes vomiting; must close her eyes while bathing (Lyss.).

Cannot talk, the larynx is so painful; is dry, raw, rough, sore.

Cough: Going from warm to cold air (reverse of Bry.); < from laughing, talking, reading, drinking, eating, *lying on the left side* (Dros., Stann.).

Perspiration has the odor of sulphur.

Necrosis of the (left) lower jaw.

Relationship

Complementary: Arsenicum, with which it is isomorphic; All-c., its vegetable analogue.

Incombatible: With Causticum, must not be used before or after.

Phos. removes the bad effects of iodine and *excessive use of table salt.*

Follows well: After, Calc. or Chin.

Hahnemann says: "Acts most beneficially when patient suffers from chronic loose stool or diarrhea.

Aggravation

Evening, before midnight (Puls., Rhus-t.); *lying on left or painful side; during a thunderstorm;* weather changes, either hot or cold.

Cold air relieves the head and face symptoms but aggravates those of chest, throat and neck.

Amelioration

In the dark; lying on right side; from being rubbed or mesmerized; from cold food, cold water, until it gets warm.

PHYSOSTIGMA

Calabar Bean   *Leguminosae*

Uncommon mental activity; *cannot stop thinking.*
Vision dim; from blur or film; objects mixed.

Pain after using eyes; floating black spots, flashes of light, twitching of lids and muscles of eyes (Agar.); nystagmus.

Great prostration of muscular system; impaired locomotion (Gels.).

Tremors or trembling of young persons from mental or physical disturbances.

Idiopathic or traumatic tetanus; brought on or < *by slightest breath of air from a person passing* (Hyper., Lyss., Nux-v., Strych.).

Relationship

Compare: Bell., Con., Cur., Gels., Hyper., Strych.

PHYTOLACCA DECANDRA

Poke Root *Phytolaccaceae*

Patients of a rheumatic diathesis; rheumatism of fibrous and periosteal tissue; mercurial or syphilitic.

Emaciation, chlorosis; loss of fat.

Great exhaustion and profound prostration.

Occupies a position between Bryonia and Rhus-t.; cures when these fail though apparently well indicated.

In rheumatism and neuralgia after diphtheria, gonorrhea, mercury or syphilis.

Pain flying like electric shocks; shooting, lancinating; rapidly shifting (Lac-c., Puls.); worse from motion and at night.

PHYTOLACCA DECANDRA

Entire indifference to life; sure she will die.

Vertigo: When rising from bed feels faint (Bry.).

Intense headache and backache; lame, sore, bruised feeling all over; constant desire to move but motion < pains (Lac-c., Merc.; motion >, Rhus-t.).

Irresistible desire to bite the teeth or gums together (Pod.); during dentition.

Sore throat; of a dark-red color; uvula large, dropsical, almost translucent (Kali-bi., Rhus-t.).

Diphtheria: Pains shoot from throat into ears on swallowing; great pain at root of tongue when swallowing; *burning, as from a coal on fire or a red-hot iron; dryness;* difficult to swallow with trembling of the hands; sensation of a lump in the throat with continuous desire to swallow; tonsils, uvula and back part of throat covered with ash-colored membrane; *cannot drink hot fluids* (Lach.).

Carotid and submaxillary glands indurated after diphtheria, scarlet fever.

Mammae full of hard, painful nodosites.

Breast, shows an early tendency *to cake;* **is full, stony, hard and painful,** especially when suppuration in inevitable; when child nurses pain goes *from nipple all over body* (goes to back, Crot-t.; to uterus, Puls., Sil.).

Mammary abscess; *fistula, gaping, angry ulcers;* pus sanious, ichorous, fetid; unhealthy.

Tumefied breast neither heals nor suppurates, is of a purple hue and "hard as old cheese" (Bry., Lac-c., Phel.).

Nipples, sensitive, *sore, fissured* (Graph.); < intensely by nursing, pain radiates over whole body.

Hasten suppuration (Hep., Lach., Merc., Sil.).

Relationship

Compare: Kali-i., its analogue.

Aggravation

When it rains; exposure to damp, cold weather.

PICRICUM ACIDUM

Picric Acid $HC_6H_2(NO_2)_3O$

Is often restorative of a washed and worn-out system; a fair picture of "nervous prostration" (Kali-p.).

Progressive, pernicious anemia; *neurasthenia.*

Brain fag: Of literary or business people; slightest excitement, mental exertion or overwork brings on headache, and causes burning along the spine (Kali-p.).

Headache: Of students; teachers and overworked businessmen; from grief or depressing emotions; *in occipital-cervical region* (Nat-m., Sil.); < or brought on by slightest motion or *mental exertion.*

Priapism, with spinal disease; erections violent, long-lasting; profuse seminal emissions; satyriasis (Canth., Phos.).

Small boils in any part of body, but not especially in external auditory canal.

Burning along spine and great weakness of spine and back; softening of cord (Phos., Zinc.).

Weariness, progressing from a slight feeling of fatigue on motion to complete paralysis.

Tired heavy feeling all over body, especially of limbs, < on exertion.

Relationship

Compare: Arg-n., Gels., Kali-p., Ph-ac., Phos., Petr., Sil.

Aggravation

Least *mental exertion;* motion; study; wet weather.

Amelioration

From cold air and cold water.

PLATINUM

Platina   *The Metal*

Adapted to women, dark hair, rigid fibre; thin, of a sanguine temperament; who suffer from too early and too profuse menses.

Sexual organs *exceedingly sensitive; cannot bear the napkin to touch her;* will go into spasms from an examination; vulva painfully sensitive during coitus; will faint during, or cannot endure coitus (compare, Murx., Orig.).

The pains increase gradually and as gradually decrease (Stann.); are attended with numbness of parts (Cham.).

For hysterical patients, alternately gay and sad, who cry easily (Croc., Ign., Puls.); pale, easily fatigued.

Arrogant, proud, contemptuous, and haughty; pitiful "looking down" upon people usually venerated; a kind of "casting them off" unwillingly.

Mental delusions, as if everything about her were small; all persons physically and mentally inferior, but she is physically large and superior.

Sensation of growing larger in every direction.

Trifling things produce profound vexation (Ign., Staph.); remains a long time in the sulks.

Satiety of life, with taciturnity and fear of death (Acon., Ars.).

Mental disturbances after fright, grief, vexation; onanism, pride.

Mental symptoms appear as physical symptoms disappear and *vice versa.*

Headache: Numb, heavy pain in brain or on vertex; from anger or chagrin; hysterical, from uterine disease; pains gradually increase and decrease.

Nymphomania; < in lying-in women; excessive *sexual development,* especially in virgins (Kali-p.); vaginismus, spasms and constriction.

Menses too early, too profuse, too long-lasting; *dark,*

clotted, offensive, with bearing-down spasms, pains in uterus with twitching; genitals sensitive.

Excessive itching in uterus; pruritus vulvae.

Constipation: While travelling (at sea, Bry.); after lead poisoning; from inertia of bowels; frequent, unsuccessful urging; *stools adhere to rectum and anus* like soft clay (Alum.); of emigrants; of pregnancy; obstinate cases after Nux has failed.

Metrorrhagia: Flow in black clots and fluid; thick, black, tarry or in a grumous mass (Croc.).

Relationship

Compare: Aur., Croc., Ign., Kali-p., Puls., Sep., Stann., Valer. the vegetable analogue.

PLUMBUM

Lead　　　　　　　　　　　　　　　　　　*The Metal*

Adapted to diseases from spinal origin (Phos., Pic-ac., Zinc.).

Excessive and rapid emaciation; general or partial paralysis; extreme, with anemia and great weakness.

Muscular atrophy from sclerosis of spinal system.

Lassitude; faints on going into a room full of company.

Slow of perception; intellectual torpor, gradually increasing apathy (in fevers, Ph-ac.).

PLUMBUM 251

Weakness or loss of memory; unable to find the proper word (Anac., Lac-c.).

Delirium alternating with colic.

Assumes strangest attitudes and positions in bed.

Complexion: *Pale, ash-colored, yellow, corpse-like, cheeks sunken;* expressive of great anxiety and suffering.

Skin of face, grease, shiny (Nat-m., Sanic.).

Distinct blue line along margin of gums; gums swollen, pale, show a lead-colored line.

Excessive pain in abdomen, *radiating to all parts of body.*

Sensation in abdomen at night, which causes patient to stretch violently for hours; must stretch in every direction (Aml-ns.).

Violent colic, sensation as if abdominal wall was drawn as if by a string to the spine.

Intussusception, with colic and fecal vomiting; strangulated hernia, femoral, inguinal or umbilical.

Constipation: *Stools hard, lumpy, black like sheep dung* (Chel., Op.); with urging and terrible pain from *spasm of anus;* obstructed evacuation and indurated feces, dryness of the excretions, paralysis or muscular atony; during pregnancy; from impaction of feces; when Platinum fails.

Bright's disease: Colic pain; abdomen retracted; rapid emaciation; excessive debility; contracted kidney.

Feels a lack of room for fetus in uterus; inability of uterus to expand; threatening abortion.

Spasms: Clonic; tonic; from cerebral sclerosis or tumor; epilepsy or epileptiform convulsions.

Yellow skin: Dark brown "liver spots" in climacteric years; jaundice, the eyes, skin and urine yellow.

Relationship

Compare: Alum., Plat., Op. in colic; Podo. in retraction of navel; Nux-v., in strangulated hernia; Podo, the vegetable analogue.

The bad effects of Plumbum are antidoted by Alum., Petr., Plat., Sul-ac., Zinc.

Aggravation

At night (pain in limbs).

Amelioration

Rubbing; hard pressure.

PODOPHYLLUM

May Apple *Berberidaceae*

Adapted to persons of bilious temperament who suffer from gastro-intestinal derangement, especially after abuse of mercury, "bilious attacks."

Thirst for large quantities of cold water (Bry.).

Pains: Sudden shocks of jerking pains.

Depression of spirits, imagines he is going to die or be very ill (Ars.); disgust for life.

PODOPHYLLUM

Headache alternates with diarrhea (Aloe); headache in winter, diarrhea in summer.

Painless cholera morbus; cholera infantum (Phyt.).

Violent cramps in feet, calves; thighs; with watery, painless stools.

Difficult dentition; moaning, grinding the teeth at night; intense desire to press the gums together (Phyt.); *head hot and rolling from side to side* (Bell., Hell.).

Diarrhea: Of long standing; *early in morning*, continues through forenoon, followed by natural stool in evening (Aloe), and accompanied by sensation of weakness of sinking in abdomen or rectum.

Diarrhea of children: During teething; after eating; *while being bathed or washed; of dirty water soaking napkin through* (Benz-ac.); with gagging.

Stool: Green, *watery, fetid, profuse* (Calc.); gushing out (Gamb., Jat., Phos.); chalk-like, jelly-like (Aloe), undigested (Chin., Ferr.); yellow meal-like sediment; prolapse of rectum before or with stool.

Prolapsus uteri: *From over-lifting or straining;* from constipation; after parturition; with subinvolution.

In early months of pregnancy, can lie comfortably, only on stomach (Acet-ac.).

Patient is *constantly rubbing and shaking the region of liver with his hand.*

Fever paroxysms at 7 a.m. with *great loquacity during chill and heat;* sleep during perspiration.

Affects right throat, right ovary, right hypochondrium (Lyc.).

Pain and numbness in right ovary, running down thigh of that side (Lil-t.).

Suppressed menses in young girls (Puls., Tub.).

Relationship

Compare: Aloe, Chel., Coll., Lil-t., Merc., Nux-v., Sulph.

It antidotes the bad effects of mercury.

After: Ip., Nux-v., in gastric affections; after Calc. and Sulph. in liver diseases.

Aggravation

In early morning (Aloe, Nux-v., Sulph.); in hot weather; during dentition.

PSORINUM

A Product of Psora *A Nosode*

Especially adapted to the psoric constitution.

In chronic cases *when well selected remedies fail to relieve or permanently improve* (in acute diseases, Sulph.); when Sulphur seems indicated but fails to act.

Lack of reaction after severe acute diseases. Appetite will not return.

Children are pale, delicate, sickly. Sick babies will not sleep day or night but worry, fret, cry (Jal.); child is good, plays all day; restless, troublesome, screaming all night (reverse of Lyc.).

PSORINUM

Great weakness and debility: From loss of animal fluids; *remaining after acute diseases,* independent of or without any organic lesion, or apparent cause.

Body has a filthy smell, even after bathing.

The whole body is painful, *easily sprained and injured.*

Great sensitiveness to cold air *or change of weather;* wears a fur cap, overcoat or shawl even in hottest summer weather.

Stormy weather he feels acutely restless for days before or during a thunderstorm (Phos.); dry, scaly eruptions *disappear in summer, return in winter.*

Ailments: From suppressed itch or other skin diseases, when Sulphur fails to relieve; severe, from even slight emotions.

Feels unusually well day before attack.

Extremely psoric patients; nervous, restless, easily startled.

All excretions—diarrhea, leucorrhea, menses, perspiration—**have a carrion-like odor.**

Anxious, full of fear; evil forebodings.

Religious melancholy: Very depressed, sad suicidal thoughts; despairs of salvation (Meli.), of recovery.

Despondent: Fears he will die; that he will fail in business; during climaxis; making his own life and that of those about him intolerable.

Driven to despair with excessive itching.

Headache: Preceded, by flickering before eyes, by dimness of vision or blindness (Lac-d., Kali-bi.), by black spots or rings.

Headache: *Always hungry during; > while eating* (Anac., Kali-p.); from suppressed eruptions, or suppressed menses; > nosebleed (Meli.).

Hair, dry lusterless, tangles easily, glues together (Lyc.). Plica polonica (Bar., Sars., Tub.).

Scalp: Dry, scaly or moist, (fetid, suppurating eruptions; oozing a sticky, offensive fluid Graph., Mez.).

Intense photophobia, with inflamed lids; cannot open the eyes; lies with face buried in pillow.

Ears: Humid scurfs and soreness on and behind ears; oozing an offensive viscid fluid (Graph.).

Otorrhea: Thin, ichorous, horribly fetid discharge, like decayed meat; chronic, after measles or scarlatina.

Acne: All forms, simplex, rosacea; < during menses, from coffee, fats, sugar, meat; when the best selected remedy fails or only palliates.

Hungry in the middle of the night; must have something to eat (Cina, Sulph.).

Eructations tasting of rotten eggs (Arn., Ant-t., Graph.).

Quinsy, tonsils greatly swollen, difficult, painful swallowing; burns, feels scalded; cutting, tearing, intense pain to ears on swallowing (painless, Bar-c.); profuse, offensive saliva; tough mucus in throat, must hawk continually, to not only > acute attack but *eradicate the tendency.*

Hawks up cheesy balls, size of pea, of disgusting taste and carrion-like odor (Kali-m.).

Diarrhea: Sudden, imperative (Aloe, Sulph.); stool watery, dark brown, *fetid; smells like carrion;* involuntary,

< at night from 1 to 4 a.m.; after severe acute diseases; teething; in children; when weather changes.

Constipation: Obstinate, with backache; from inactivity of rectum; when Sulphur fails to relieve.

Enuresis: From vesical paresis; during full moon, obstinate cases, with a family history of eczema.

Chronic gonorrhea of year's duration that can neither be suppressed nor cured; the best selected remedy fails.

Leucorrhea: Large, clotted lumps of an intolerable odor; violent pains in sacrum; debility; during climaxis.

During pregnancy: Most obstinate vomiting, fetus moves too violently; when the best selected remedy fails to relieve; to correct the psoric diathesis of the unborn.

Profuse perspiration after acute diseases, *with relief of all suffering* (Calad., Nat-m.).

Asthma, dyspnea; < in open air, sitting up (Laur.); > *lying down* and keeping arms stretched far apart (reverse of, Ars.); despondent, thinks he will die.

Cough returns every winter.

Hay fever: Appearing regularly every year the same day of the month; with an asthmatic, psoric or eczematous history. Patient should be treated the previous winter to eradicate the diathesis and prevent summer attack.

Cough: After suppressed itch, or eczema; chronic, of year's duration < mornings on waking and evenings on lying down (Phos., Tub.); sputa green, yellow or salty mucus; pus-like; coughs a long time before expectorating.

Skin: Abnormal tendency to receive skin diseases (Sulph.); eruptions easily suppurate (Hep.); *dry, inactive, rarely sweats; dirty look*, as if never washed; coarse, greasy, as if bathed in oil; bad effects from suppression by sulphur and zinc ointments.

Sleepless from intolerable itching, or frightful dreams of robbers, danger, etc. (Nat-m.).

Psorinum should not be given for psora or the psoric diathesis, but like every other remedy, upon a strict individualization—the totality of the symptoms and then we realize its wonderful work.

Relationship

Complementary: Sulphur and Tuberculinum.

Is followed well: By, Alum., Borx., Hep., Sulph., Tub.

After: Lac-ac., in vomiting of pregnancy.

After Arn. in traumatic affections of ovaries.

Sulphur follows Psorinum well in mammary cancer.

"Whether derived from purest gold or purest filth, our gratitude for its excellent service forbids us to inquire or care.— P.B. Bell.

PULSATILLA

Anemone   *Ranunculaceae*

Adapted to persons of indecisive, slow, phlegmatic temperament; sandy hair, blue eyes, pale face, easily moved to laughter or tears; affectionate, mild, gentle, timid, yielding disposition—the woman's remedy.

Weeps easily: Almost impossible to detail her ailments without weeping (weeps when thanked, Lyc.).

Especially in diseases of women and children.

Women inclined to be fleshy, with *scanty and protracted menstruation* (Graph.).

The first serious impairment of health is referred to puberic age, have "never been well since"—anemia, chlorosis, bronchitis, phthisis.

Secretions from all mucous membranes *are thick, bland and yellowish-green* (Kali-s., Nat-s.).

Symptoms ever changing; no two chills, no two stools, no two attacks alike; very well one hour, very miserable the next; apparently contradictory (Ign.).

Pains: Drawing, tearing, erratic, **rapidly shifting** *from one part to another* (Kali-bi., Lac-c., Mang-act.); are accompanied with constant chilliness; the more severe the pain, the more severe the chill; appear suddenly, leave gradually, or tension much increases until very acute and then "lets up with a snap"; on first motion (Rhus-t.).

Thirstlessness *with nearly all complaints;* gastric difficulties from eating rich food, cake, pastry, especially after pork or sausage; the sight or even the thought of pork cases disgust; "bad taste" in the morning.

Great dryness of mouth in the morning, without thirst (Nux-m.; mouth moist, intense thirst, Merc.).

Mumps; metastasis to mammae or testicle.

"All-gone" sensation in stomach, in tea drinkers especially.

Diarrhea: Only, or usually *at night;* watery, greenish-yellow, *very changeable;* soon as they eat; from fruit, cold food or drinks, ice-cream (Ars., Bry.; eating pears, Verat., Chin.; onions, Thuja; oysters, Brom., Lyc.; milk, Calc., Nat-c., Nicc., Sulph.; drinking impure water, Camph., Zing.).

Derangements at puberty; menses, suppressed from getting the feet wet; *too late,* scanty, slimy, painful, irregular, *intermittent flow,* with evening chilliness; with intense pain and great restlessness and tossing about (Mag-p.); *flows more during day* (on lying down, Kreos.). Delayed first menstruation.

Sleep: Wide awake in the evening, does not want to go to bed; first sleep restless, sound asleep when it is time to get up; awakes languid, unrefreshed (reverse of, Nux-v.).

Styes: Especially on upper lid; *from eating fat, greasy, rich food or pork* (compare, Lyc., Staph.).

Threatened abortion; flow ceases and then returns with increased force; pains spasmodic, excite suffocation and fainting; must have fresh air.

Toothache: Relieved by holding cold water in the mouth (Bry., Coff.); worse form warm things and heat of room.

Unable to breathe well, or is chilly in warm room.

Nervousness, intensely felt about the ankles.

Relationship

Complementary: Kali-m., Lyc., Sil., Sul-ac.; Kali-m. is its chemical analogue.

Silicea is the chronic of Pulsatilla in nearly all ailments.

Follows, and is followed by, Kali-m.

One of the best remedies with which to begins the treatment of a chronic case (Calc., Sulph.).

Patients, anemic or chlorotic, who have taken much iron, quinine and tonics, even years before.

Ailments: From abuse of chamomile, quinine, mercury, tea drinking, sulphur.

Follows well: After, Kali-bi., Lyc., Sep., Sil., Sulph.

Aggravation

In a warm close room; evening, at twilight; on beginning to move; lying on the left, or *on the painless side;* very rich, fat, indigestible food; pressure on the well side if it be made toward the diseased side; warm applications; *heat* (Kali-m.).

Amelioration

In the open air; lying on painful side (Bry.); cold air or cool room; eating or drinking cold things; cold applications (Kali-m.).

PYROGENIUM

A Product of Sepsis   *A Nosode*

For sapremia or septicemia; puerperal or surgical from ptomaine or sewer gas infection; during course of diphtheria, typhoid or typhus; *when the best selected remedy fails to > or permanently improve.*

The bed feels hard (Arn.); *parts lain on feel sore and bruised* (Bapt.); rapid decubitis (Carb-ac.).

Great restlessness; must move constantly to > the soreness of parts (Arn., Eup-per.).

Tongue: *Large, flabby;* **clean, smooth as if vanished; fiery red;** dry, cracked, articulation difficult (Crot-h., Ter.).

Taste: *Sweetish; terribly fetid;* **pus-like;** as from an abscess.

Vomiting: Persistent; brownish, coffee-ground; offensive, stercoraceous; with impacted or obstructed bowels (Op., Plb.).

Diarrhea: Horribly offensive (Psor.); brown or black (Lept.); painless, involuntary; uncertain, when passing flatus (Aloe, Olnd.).

Constipation: With complete inertia (Op., Sanic.); *obstinate from impaction, in fevers;* **stool, large, black, carrion-like;** *small black balls,* like olives (Op., Plb.).

Fetus: Or secundines retained, decomposed; dead for days, black; horribly offensive discharge; "never well since" septic fever, following abortion or confinement. To arouse vital activity of uterus.

Lochia: Thin, acrid, brown, very fetid (Nit-ac.); suppressed, followed by chills, fever and profuse fetid perspiration.

Distinct consciousness of a heart; it feels tired; as if enlarged; purring, throbbing, pulsating, constant in ears, preventing sleep; cardiac asthenia from septic conditions.

Pulse abnormally rapid, out of all proportion to temperature (Lil-t.).

Skin; pale, cold, of an ashy hue (Sec.); obstinate, varicose, offensive ulcers of old persons (Psor.).

Chill: *Begins in the back,* between scapulae; severe, *general, of bones and extremities;* marking onset of septic fever; temperature 103 to 106; heat sudden, skin dry and burning; pulse rapid, small, wiry, 140 to 170; cold clammy sweat follows.

In septic fevers, especially puerperal—Pyrogenium has demonstrated its great value as a homoeopathic dynamic antiseptic.

Relationship

Compare: Ars., Carb-v., Carb-ac., Op., Psor., Rhus-t., Sec., Verat.

Latent pyrogenic process, patient continually relapsing after apparent simillimum.

RATANHIA

Rhatany *Polygalaceae*

Terrible toothache during early months of pregnancy; tooth feels elongated; < *lying,* compelling to rise and walk about.

Constipation: Stool hard *with great straining;* protrusion of hemorrhoids followed by long-lasting aching and *burning in anus* (Sulph.); bowels inactive; pain after stool as if *splinters of glass* were sticking in anus and rectum (Thuj).

Excruciating pains after stool; burning after soft stool (Nit-ac.).

Fissures of anus, great sensitiveness of rectum.

Fissures of nipples in nursing women (Graph., Sep.).

Relationship

Compare: Canth., Carb-ac., Iris, Sulph., Thuj.

RANUNCULUS BULBOSUS

Buttercup   *Ranunculaceae*

One of our most effective remedies for *the bad effects of alcoholic beverages;* spasmodic hicough; delirium tremens.

Day blindness; mist before eyes; pressure and smarting in eyeballs (Phos.).

Muscular pain about margins of shoulder blades in women of sedentary employment, often burning in small spots (Agar., Phos.); from needlework, typewriting, piano playing (Cimic.).

Pains: *Stitches, sharp, smoothing, neuralgic, myalgic or rheumatic in walls of chest,* coming in paroxysms; excited or brought on by atmospheric changes; inflammatory; depending upon spinal irritation (Agar.).

Pleurisy or pneumonia from sudden exposure to cold, while overheated, or *vice versa* (Acon., Arn.).

Corns sensitive to touch, smart, burn (Sal-ac.).

Intercostal rheumatism; **chest sore, bruised < from touch, motion or turning the body** (Bry.); in wet, stormy weather (Rhus-t.).

Shingles preceded or followed by intercostal neuralgia (Mez.); vesicles may have a bluish appearance.

Relationship

Compare: Acon., Arn., Bry., Clem., Euphorbia., Mez.

Incompatible: With Sulph. and Staph.

Aggravation

Contact; motion atmospheric changes, especially, wet stormy weather (Rhus-t.).

RHEUM

Rhubarb   *Polygonaceae*

Suitable for children, especially during dentition.

Sour smell of the whole body; child smells sour, even after washing or bathing (Hep., Mag-c.).

Screaming of children with urging and sour stools.

Children cry and toss about all night (Psor.).

Child impatient, desires many things, and cries; dislikes even favorite play things (Cina, Staph.).

Sweat of scalp, constant, profuse; whether asleep or awake, quiet or in motion, the hair is always wet; may or may not be sour (Calc., Sanic.).

Difficult dentition; child restless, irritable, peevish, with pale face and sour smell (Kreos., Cham.).

Desires various kinds of food, but cannot eat them; becomes repugnant.

Colic: < at once by uncovering an arm or leg; *with very sour stool;* < when standing; not > by stool.

Relationship

Complementary: After Mag-c., when milk disagrees and child has a sour odor.

Compare: Cham., Coloc., Hep., Ip., Mag-c., Podo., Staph., Sulph.

May be given after abuse of Magnesia, with or without rhubarb, if stools are sour.

RHODODENDRON

Snowrose *Ericaceae*

Nervous persons *who dread a storm* and are particularly afraid of thunder; < before the storm, especially an electrical storm (Nat-c., Phos., Psor., Sil.).

Toothache, every spring and fall during sharp east winds; worse from *change of weather, thunderstorm,* **windy weather.**

Acute inflammatory swelling of joints, wandering

from one joint to another; severe at night; < in rest and during rough stormy weather (Kalm.).

Rheumatic drawing, tearing pains in all the limbs, *worse at rest and in wet, cold, windy weather* (Rhus-t.).

Cannot get asleep or remain asleep unless legs are crossed.

Gout with fibrous deposit in great toe joint, rheumatic, often mistaken for bunion (Colch., Led.).

Induration and swelling of the testicle after gonorrhea or rheumatic exposure (Clem.); orchitis, sensation in gland as if it were being crushed (Aur., Cham.).

Relationship

Compare: Bry., Con., Calc., Led., Lyc., Sep., Rhus-t.

Aggravation

Stormy, windy weather; electrical changes in the atmosphere; on approach of thunderstorm; symptoms reappear with rough weather.

Amelioration

Better from wrapping the head warmly; dry heat and exercise.

RHUS TOXICODENDRON

Poison Oak   *Anacardiaceae*

Adapted to persons of rheumatic diathesis; bad effects of getting wet, especially after being over-heated.

Ailments: From spraining or straining *a single part,* muscle or tendon (Calc., Nux-v.); overlifting, particularly from stretching high up to reach things; lying on damp ground; too much summer bathing in lake or river.

Affects the fibrous tissue, especially (Rhod.; serous, Bry.); the right side more than the left.

Pains: As if sprained; as if a muscle or tendon was torn from its attachment; as if bones were scraped with a knife; worse after midnight and in wet, rainy weather; affected parts sore to touch.

Lameness, stiffness and pain on first moving after rest, or on getting up in the morning, > by walking or continued motion.

Great restlessness, anxiety, apprehension (Acon., Ars.); cannot remain in bed, must change position often to obtain relief from pain (from mental anxiety, Ars.).

Restless, cannot stay long in one position.

Back: Pain between the shoulders on swallowing; pain and stiffness in small of back < sitting or lying, > by motion or lying on something hard.

Great sensitiveness *to open air*; putting the hand from under the bed-cover brings on cough (Bar-c., Hep.).

Muscular rheumatism, sciatica, left side (Coloc.); aching in left arm, with heart disease.

Great apprehension at night; fears he will die of being poisoned; cannot remain in bed.

Vertigo, when standing or walking; worse when

lying down (better when lying down, Apis); < rising from lying, or stooping (Bry.).

Headache: Brain feels loose when stepping or shaking the head; sensation of swashing in brain; stupefying; as if torn; *from beer;* returns from least chagrin; < from sitting, lying, in cold, > warmth and motion.

Dreams of great exertion; rowing, swimming, working hard at his daily occupation (Bry.).

Corners of mouth ulcerated, fever blisters around mouth and on chin (Nat-m.).

Tongue: Dry, sore, red, cracked; **triangular red tip;** takes imprint of teeth (Chel., Podo.).

Great thirst, with dry tongue, mouth and throat.

External genitals inflamed, erysipelatous, edematous.

A dry, teasing cough, before and during chill, in intermittent fever; cough, with taste of blood.

When acute diseases assume a typhoid form.

Diarrhea: *With beginning typhoid;* involuntary, *with great exhaustion;* tearing pain down the posterior part of limbs during stool.

Paralysis: With numbness of affected parts; from getting wet on lying on damp ground; after exertion, parturition, sexual excesses, ague or typhoid; paresis of limbs; ptosis.

Erysipelas, from left to right; *vesicular,* yellow vesicles; much swelling, inflammation; burning, itching, stinging.

Relationship

Complementary: To, Bryonia.

Inimical: To, Apis, must not be used before or after.

Compare: Arn., Bry., Rhod., Nat-s., Sulph.

Aggravation

Before a storm; *cold, wet rainy weather;* at night, especially after midnight; from getting wet while perspiring; *during rest.*

Amelioration

Warm, dry weather, wrapping up; warm or hot things; *motion; change of position; moving affected parts.*

The great characteristic of Rhus-t. is that with few exceptions the pains occur and are < *during repose and are* > *by motion.*

Sepia, often quickly > itching and burning of Rhus-t., the vesicles drying up in a few days.

Rhus-t. is best antidoted by the simillimum; the potentized remedy given internally. The dermatitis should never by treated by topical medicated applications; they only suppress, never cure.

RUMEX CRISPUS

Yellow Dock *Polygonaceae*

For the tubercular diathesis, extremely sensitive skin and mucous membranes.

RUMEX CRISPUS

Extremely sensitive to open air; hoarseness; worse evening; after exposure to cold; voice uncertain.

Tickling in throat pit, causing dry, teasing cough.

Dry, incessant, fatiguing cough; **worse form changing air or room** (Phos., Spong.); evening after lying down; touching or pressing the throat pit; lying on left side (Phos.); *from* **slightest inhalation of cold air; covers head with bedclothes** *to make air warmer;* little or no expectoration.

The cough is < in cool air or by anything which increases the volume or rapidity of inspired air.

Sensation of lump in throat; descends on swallowing, but returns immediately.

Raw sensation in larynx and trachea when coughing (Caust.).

Urine; involuntary with cough (Caust., Puls., Sil.).

Early morning diarrhea; from 5 to 10 a.m. (Aloe, Nat-s., Podo., Sulph.); stools painless, profuse, offensive; sudden urging, driving out of bed in morning.

Skin: Itching of various parts; < by cold, > by warmth; *when undressing, uncovering or exposing to cold air* (Hep., Nat-s., Olnd.).

Relationship

Compare: Bell., Caust., Dros., Hyos., Phos., Sang., Sulph.

Aggravation

Cool or cold air; lying down (Hyos.).

Amelioration

Warmth; *keeping mouth covered* to exclude cold air.

RUTA GRAVEOLENS

Rue   *Rutaceae*

Scrofulous exostosis; bruises and other mechanical injuries of bones and periosteum; sprains; periostitis; erysipelas; fractures, and especially dislocations (Symph.).

Bruised lame sensation all over, as after a fall or blow; worse in limbs and joints (Arn.).

All parts of the body upon which he lies are painful, as if bruised (Bapt., Pyrog.).

Restless, turns and changes position frequently when lying (Rhus-t.).

Lameness after sprains, especially of wrists and ankles (chronic sprains, Bov., Stront.).

Phthisis after mechanical injuries to chest (Mill.).

Aching in and over eyes, with blurred vision, as if they had been strained.

After using eyes at fine work, watch making, engraving (Nat-m.); looking intently (Senec.).

Amblyopia or asthenopia from over-exertion of eyes or anomalies of refraction; from overuse in bad light; fine sewing, over-reading at night; misty, dim vision, with complete obscuration at a distance.

Eyes burn, ache, feel strained; hot, like balls of fire; spasms of lower lids.

Constipation; from inactivity, or impaction following mechanical injuries (Arn.).

Prolapse of rectum, *immediately on attempting a passage;* from the slightest stooping; after confinement; frequent unsuccessful urging.

Pressure on the bladder as if constantly full; *continues after urinating;* could hardly retain urine on account of urging, yet if not attended to it was difficult afterwards to void it; scanty green urine; involuntary.

Warts; with sore pains; flat, smooth on palms of hands (Nat-c., Nat-m. — on back of hands, Dul.).

Backache, relieved by lying on the back.

Relationship

Compare: Arn., Arg-n., Con., Euphr., Phyt., Rhus., Symph.

After Arnica, it hastens the curative process in the joints; after Symphytum, in injuries of bones.

SABADILLA

Cevadilla   *Liliaceae*

Suited to persons of light hair, fair complexion with a weak, relaxed muscular system.

Worm affections of children (Cina, Sil., Spig.).

Nervous diseases; twitching, convulsive tremblings, catalepsy; from worms (Cina, Psor.).

Illusions: That he is sick; parts shrunken; that she is pregnant when merely distended from flatus; that she has some horrible throat diseases that will be fatal.

Delirium during intermittents (Podo.).

Sneezing in spasmodic paroxysms; followed by lachrymation; copious watery coryza; face hot and eyelids red and burning.

Diphtheria, tonsillitis; *can swallow warm food more easily;* stitches and most symptoms, especially of throat, go from left to right (Lach., Lac-c.).

Sensation of a skin hanging loosely in throat, must swallow over it.

Headache: *From too much thinking,* too close application or attention (Arg-n.); from worms.

Dryness of fauces and throat.

Parchment-like dryness of skin.

Relationship

Compare: Coloc., Colch., Lyc., where < is from 4 to 8 p.m.; Puls., Sabad. > in open air.

Follows: Bry. and Ran-b. well in pleurisy, and has cured after Acon. and Bry. failed.

SABINA

Savine *Coniferae*

Chronic ailments of women; arthritic pains; tendency to miscarriages, especially at third mouth.

Music is intolerable: Produces nervousness, goes through bone and marrow (causes weeping, Thuj.).

Drawing pains in small of back, **from sacrum to pubes,** in nearly all diseases (from back, going round the body to pubes, Vib.).

Ailments: Following abortion or premature labor; hemorrhage from the uterus; flow partly pale red, partly clotted; *worse from* **least motion** (Sec.); often relieved by walking; *pain extending from sacrum to pubes.*

Menses: Too early, too profuce, too protracted; partly fluid, partly clotted (Ferr.); in persons who menstruated very early in life; flow in paroxysms; with colic and labor-like pains; *pains from sacrum to pubes.*

Discharge of blood between periods, with sexual excitement (Ambr.).

Retained placenta from atony of uterus; intense after, pains (Caul., Sec.).

Menorrhagia: During climacteric, in women who formerly aborted; with early first menses.

Inflammation of ovaries or uterus after abortion or premature labor.

Promotes expulsion of moles or foreign bodies from uterus (Canth.).

Fig warts with intolerable itching and burning; exuberant granulations (Thuj., Nit-ac.).

Relationship

Complementary: To, Thuj.
Compare: Calc., Croc., Mill., Sec., Tril-p.
Follows: Thuja in condyloma and sycotic affections.

Aggravation

From least motion (Sec.); warm air or room (Apis, Puls.).

Amelioration

In cool, open, fresh air.

SAMBUCUS NIGRA

Elder   *Caprifoliaceae*

Adapted to diseases of scrofulous children, which affect the air passages especially.

Persons formerly robust and fleshy, suddenly become emaciated (Iod., Tub.).

Bad effects of violent mental emotions; anxiety, grief, or excessive sexual indulgence (Ph-ac., Kali-p.).

Edematous swelling in various parts of the body, especially in leg, instep and feet.

Dry coryza of infants (sniffles); nose dry and completely obstructed, preventing breathing and nursing (Am-c., Nux-v.).

Dyspnea: Child awakens suddenly nearly suffocated, face livid, blue, sits up in bed; turns blue, gasps for breath, which it finally gets; attack passes off but is again repeated; **child inspires but cannot expire** (Chlorine, Meph.); sleeps into the attack (Lach.); compare, Arum-d. in Miller's asthma.

Attacks of suffocation as in last stage of croup.

Cough: Suffocative, with crying children; worse about midnight; hollow, deep whooping, with spasm of chest; with regular inhalations but signing exhalations.

Cough deep, dry, precedes the fever paroxysm.

Fever: *Dry heat while he sleeps; on falling asleep;* after lying down; without thirst, *dreads uncovering* (must be covered in every stage, Nux-v.).

Profuse sweat over entire body **during waking hours;** on going to sleep, dry heat returns (sweats as soon as he closes his eyes to sleep, Chin., Con.).

Relationship

Compare: Chin., Chlor., Ip., Meph., Sulph.

Relieves ailments from abuse of Arsenicum.

Follows well: After Opium in bad effects of fright.

Aggravation

During rest; after eating fruit.

Amelioration

Sitting up in bed. Motion; most of the pain occur during rest and disappear during motion (Rhus-t.).

SANGUINARIA

Bloodroot *Papaveraceae*

The periodical sick headache; begins in morning, increases during the day, lasts until evening; head feels as if it would burst, or as if eyes would be pressed out; *relieved by sleep.*

American sick headache, > by perfect quiet in a dark room ("tired headache" from over mental or physical exertion, Epigea; sick headache < during rest > by rubbing, pressing, motion, Indigo).

Headache *begins in occiput,* spreads upwards and settles over right eye (Sil.; over or in left orbit, Spig.).

Headaches, *return at the climacteric;* every seventh day (Sabad., Sil., Sulph.; eighth day, Iris).

Neuralgia of face > kneeling down and pressing the head firmly against the floor; pain extends in all directions from the upper jaw.

Circumscribed red cheeks in afternoon; burning in ears; in bronchitis, pneumonia, phthisis.

Rheumatic pain in *the right arm and shoulder* (left, Ferr.); cannot raise the arm, < at night.

Pains in places where the bones are least covered, as tibia, backs of hands, etc. (Rhus-v.).

Burning in pharynx and esophagus.

Laryngeal or nasal polypi (Sangin-n., Psor., Teucr.).

Climacteric ailments: Flushes of heat and leucorrhea; burning of palms and soles; compelled to throw off bedclothes; painful enlargement of breasts; when Lachesis and Sulphur fail to relieve.

Asthma after the "rose cold," < from odors.

Cough: Dry, waking him at night and not ceasing until he sits up in bed and passes flatus; *circumscribed red cheeks;* night sweats; diarrhea.

Severe cough after whooping cough; the cough returns every time the patient takes cold.

Eruption on face of young women, especially during scanty menses (Bell-p., Calc., Eug-j., Psor.).

Relationship

Compare: Bell., Iris, Mell., in sick headache; Lach., Sulph., in climacteric affections; Chel., Phos., Sulph., Verat-v., in chronic bronchitis or latent pneumonia.

After Bell. fails in scarlatina.

As a dynamic remedy for the narcosis of Opium.

SANICULA

Mineral Spring Water

Dread of downward motion (Borx.).

Child headstrong, obstinate, cries and kicks; cross, irritable, quickly alternates with laughter; does not want to be touched.

Constantly changing his occupation.

Head and neck of children sweat profusely during sleep; wets the pillow far around (Calc., Sil.).

Profuse, scaly dandruff on scalp, eyebrows, in the beard.

Soreness behind ears with discharge of white, gray, viscid fluid (Graph., Psor.).

Tongue: Large, flabby; burning, must protrude it to keep it cool; ringworm on tongue (Nat-m.).

Nausea and vomiting from car or carriage riding.

Thirst; drinks little and often; is vomited as soon as it reaches the stomach (Ars., Phos.).

Symptoms constantly changing (Lac-c., Puls.).

Incontinence of urine and feces; sphincter unreliable (Aloe); urging from flatus, must cross legs to prevent feces escaping.

Constipation: No desire until a large accumulation; after great straining stool partially expelled, recedes (Sil., Thuj.); large evacuation of small, dry, gray balls, must be removed mechanically (Sel.).

Stool: Hard, impossible to evacuate; of grayish-white balls, like burnt lime; crumbling from verge of anus (Mag-m.); with the odor of limburger cheese.

Diarrhea: Changeable in character and color; like scrambled eggs; frothy, grass-green, turns green on standing; like scum of a frog pond; after eating, must hurry from table.

The odor of stool follows despite bathing (Sulph.).

Excoriation of skin about anus (Sulph.); covering perineum and extending to genitals.

Leucorrhea with strong odor of fish brine (oozing from rectum smelling like herring brine, Calc.; fish brine discharge from ear, Tell.).

Weakness, bearing down as if contents of pelvis would escape; < walking, mis-step, or jar, > by rest, lying down; desire to support parts by placing hand against vulva (Lil-t., Murx.); soreness of uterus.

Foot sweat: Between the toes, making them sore; offensive (Graph., Psor., Sil.); on soles as if he had stepped in cold water.

Burning of soles of feet; must uncover or put them in a cool place (Lach., Med., Sang., Sulph.).

Child kicks off clothing even in coldest weather (Hep., Sulph.).

Emaciation, progressive; *child looks old, dirty, greasy and brownish;* skin about neck *wrinkled, hangs in folds* (Abrot., Iod., Nat-m., Sars.).

Relationship

Related to: Abrot., Alum., Borx., Calc., Graph., Nat-m., Sil., and others of our great anti-psorics.

SARSAPARILLA

Wild Liquorice   *Smilaceae*

For dark-haired persons, lithic or sycotic diathesis.

Great emaciation; skin becomes shriveled or lies in folds (Abrot., Iod., Nat-m., Sanic.).

Headache and periosteal pains generally from mercury, syphilis or suppressed gonorrhea.

In children; face like old people; enlarged abdomen; dry, flabby skin (Bar-c., Op.).

Herpetic eruptions on all parts of body; ulcers, after abuse of mercury, in syphilis.

Rash from exposure to open air; dry, itch-like eruptions, prone to appear in spring; become crusty.

Severe, almost unbearable pain **at conclusion of urination** (Berb., Equis., Med., Thuj.).

Passage of *gravel or small calculi; renal colic; stone in bladder; bloody urine.*

Urine: Bright and clear but irritating; *scanty, slimy, flaky, sandy, copious, passed without sensation* (Caust.); deposits while sand.

Painful distention and tenderness in bladder; urine *dribbles while sitting,* standing, passes freely; air passes from urethra.

Sand in urine or on diaper; child screams before and while passing it (Borx., Lyc.).

Gonorrhea checked by cold, wet weather, or mercury, followed by rheumatism.

Neuralgia or renal colic; excruciating pains from right kidney downwards (Lyc.).

Intolerable stench on genital organs; fluid pollutions; bloody seminal emission (Led., Merc.).

Retraction of nipples; nipples are small, withered, unexcitable (Sil.).

Rheumatism, bone pains after mercury or checked gonorrhea; pains < at night, in damp weather or after taking cold water.

Itching eruption of forehead during menses (Eug-j., Sang., Psor.).

Rhagades: Skin cracked on hands and feet; pain and burning, particularly on sides of fingers and toes; skin hard, indurated.

Relationship

Complementary: Merc., Sep., either or which follows well.

Compare: Berb., Lyc., Nat-m., Phos.

Frequently called for after abuse of mercury.

SECALE CORNUTUM

Spurred Rye, Ergot   *A Fungus, A Nosode*

Adapted to women of thin, *scrawny, feeble, cachectic appearance;* irritable, nervous temperament; pale, sunken countenance.

Very old, decrepit, feeble persons.

Women of very lax muscular fibre; *everything seems loose and open; no action; vessels flabby;* passive hemorrhages, copious flow of thin, black, watery blood; the corpuscles are destroyed.

Hemorrhagic diathesis; the slightest wound causes bleeding for weeks (Lach., Phos.); discharge of sanious liquid blood with a strong tendency to putrescence; tingling in the limbs and great debility, especially when the weakness is not caused by previous loss of fluids.

Leucorrhea; green, brown, offensive.

Boils: *Small, painful with green contents,* mature very slowly and heal in same manner, very debilitating.

Face: Pale, pinched, ashy, sunken, hippocratic; drawn, with sunken eyes; blue rings around eyes.

Unnatural, ravenous appetite; even with exhausting diarrhea; craves acids, lemonade.

Diarrhea: Profuse, watery, putrid, brown; discharged with great force (Gamb., Crot-h.); very exhausting; painless, involuntary; anus wide open (Apis, Phos.).

Enuresis: Of old people; urine pale, watery, or bloody; urine suppressed.

Burning; in all parts of the body, as if sparks of fire were falling on the patient (Ars.).

Gangrene; dry, senile, < from external heat.

Large ecchymosis; blood blisters; often commencement of gangrene.

Collapse in cholera diseases; skin cold, yet cannot bear to be covered (Camph.).

The skin feels cold to the touch, yet the patient cannot tolerate covering; icy coldness of extremities.

Menses: Irregular; copious, dark fluid; with pressing, labor-like pains in abdomen; continuous discharge of watery blood until next period.

Threatened abortion especially at third month (Sab.) prolonged, bearing down, forcing pains.

During labor: Pains irregular; too weak; feeble or ceasing; everything seems *loose and open but no expulsive action;* fainting.

After-pains: Too long; too painful; hour-glass contraction.

Suppression of milk; in thin, scrawny, exhausted women; the breasts do not properly fill.

Pulse small, rapid, contracted and often intermittent.

Relationship

Compare: Cinnamomum in post-partum hemorrhage; it increases labor pains, controls profuse or dangerous flooding, is always safe, while Ergot is always dangerous.

Similar: To Arsenicum, but cold and heat are opposite.

Resembles Colchicum in cholera morbus.

Aggravation

Heat; warmth from covering, of all affected parts, in all diseases *worse from heat.*

Amelioration

In the cold air; getting cold uncovering affected facted parts; rubbing.

SELENIUM

Selenium   *The Element*

Adapted to light complexion; blondes; great emaciation of face, hands, legs and feet, or single parts.

Very forgetful in business, but during sleep dreams of what he had forgotten.

Headache: Of drunkards; after debauchery; after lemonade, tea, wine; every afternoon.

Hair falls off, on head, eyebrows, whiskers, genitals.

Coryza ending in diarrhea.

Hungry: At night (Cina, Psor.); *longing for spirituous liquors,* an almost irresistible maniacal desire.

Constipation: Stool *large,* hard, impacted *so that it requires mechanical aid* (Aloe, Calc., Sanic., Sep., Sil.); after serious illness, especially enteric fevers.

Urine: Red, dark, scanty; coarse, red, sandy, sediment, involuntary dribbling while walking.

Impotence, with desire; lewd thoughts, but physically impotent (sudden impotence, Chlor.).

Erections slow, insufficient, too rapid emission with long-continued thrill; weak, ill-humored after coitus, often involuntary dribbling of semen and prostatic fluid which oozes while sitting at stool, during sleep; gleet (Calad.).

Priapism, *glands drawn up* (Berb.; drawn down, Canth.).

Aphonia: *After long use of voice;* husky when beginning to sing; obliged to clear the throat frequently of a transparent starchy mucus (Arg-m., Stann.); tubercular laryngitis.

Weak, easily exhausted; from either mental or physical labor; after typhoid, typhus, debauchery.

Irresistible desire to lie down and sleep; strength suddenly leaves him; especially in hot weather.

Very great aversion to draft of air either warm, cold or damp.

After typhoid great weakness of spine, fears paralysis.

Emaciation of affected parts.

Relationship

Compare: Phos. in genito-urinary and respiratory symptoms; Arg-met. and Stann. in laryngitis of singers or speakers; Alum., hard stool, inactive rectum.

Follows well: After, Calad., Nat-m., Staph., Ph-ac., in sexual weakness.

Itch checked by mercurials or sulphur often requires Selenium.

Aggravation

Draft of air; in the sun; from lemonade, *tea or wine.*

Amelioration

Taking cold water or cold air into the mouth.

SEPIA

Cuttle Fish *Mollusca*

Adapted to persons of dark hair, rigid fibre, but mild and easy disposition (Puls.).

Diseases of women: Especially those occurring during pregnancy; childbed and lactation; or diseases attended with sudden prostration and sinking faintness (Murx., Nux-m.); "the washerwoman's remedy," complaints that are brought on by or aggravated after laundry work.

Pains extend from other parts *to the back* (reverse of, Sab.); are attended with shuddering (with chilliness, Puls.).

Particularly sensitive to cold air, "chills so easily"; lack of vital heat, especially in chronic diseases (in acute diseases, Led.).

Sensation of a ball in inner parts; during menses, pregnancy, lactation; with constipation, diarrhea, hemorrhoids, leucorrhea and all uterine affections.

Faints easily: After getting wet; from extremes of heat or cold; riding in a carriage; while kneeling at church.

Coldness of the vertex with headache (Verat.; heat of vertex, Calc., Graph., Sulph.).

Anxiety: With fear, flushes of heat over face and head; about real or imaginary evils; towards evening.

Great sadness and weeping. Dread of being alone, of men; of meeting friends; with uterine troubles.

Indifferent: Even to one's family; to one's occupation (Fl-ac., Ph-ac.); *to those whom she loves best.*

Greedy, miserly (Lyc.).

Indolent: Does not want to do anything, either work or play; even an exertion to think.

Headache: In terrific shocks; *at menstrual nisus, with scanty flow;* in delicate, sensitive, hysterical women; pressing, bursting < motion, stooping, mental labor, > by external pressure, continued hard motion.

Great falling of the hair, after chronic headaches or at the climacteric.

Yellowness: Of the face; conjunctiva; yellow spots on the chest; *a yellow saddle across upper part of the cheeks and nose;* a "tell tale face" of uterine ailments.

All the coverings of the neck felt too tight and were constantly loosened (Lach.).

Herpes circinatus *in isolated spots* on upper part of body (in intersecting rings over whole body, Tell.).

Pot-belliedness of mothers (of children, Sulph.).

Painful sensation *of emptiness*, "all-gone feeling," in the epigastrium, relieved by eating (Chel., Murx., Phos.).

Tongue foul, but becomes clear at each menstrual nisus, returns when flow ceases; swelling and cracking of lower lip.

Constipation: During pregnancy (Alum.); stool hard, knotty, in balls, insufficient, difficult; pain in rectum during and long after stool (Nit-ac., Sulph.); sense of weight or ball in anus, not > by stool.

Urine: Deposits a reddish clay-colored sediment which adheres to the vessel as if it had been burned on; fetid, so offensive must be removed from the room (horribly offensive after standing, Indium).

Enuresis: Bed is wet almost as soon as the child goes to sleep (Kreos.); always during *the first sleep*.

Gleet: Painless, yellowish, staining linen; meatus glued together in morning; obstinate, of long standing (Kali-i.); sexual organs, weak and exhausted.

Violent stitches upward in the vagina; lancinating pains from the uterus to the umbilicus.

Prolapsus of uterus and vagina; **pressure and bearing down as if everything would protrude from pelvis;** must cross limbs tightly or "sit close" to prevent it; with oppression of breathing (compare Agar., Bell., Lil-t., Murx., Sanic.).

Irregular menses of nearly every form—early, late, scanty, profuse, amenorrhea or menorrhagia—when associated with above named symptoms.

Morning sickness of pregnancy; the sight or thought of food sickens (Nux-v.); the smell of cooking food nauseates (Ars., Colch.).

Dyspnea; < sitting, after sleep, in room, > dancing or walking rapidly.

Erythism; flushes of heat from least motion; with anxiety and faintness; followed by perspiration over whole body; *climacteric* (Lach., Sang., Sulph., Tub.); *ascends,* from pelvic organs.

Itching of skin; of various parts; of external genitalia; is not > by scratching, and is apt to change to burning (Sulph.).

Relationship

Complementary: Natrium mur.

Inimical: To Lach., should not be used before or after; to, Puls., with which it should never be alternated.

Similar: To, Lach., Sang., Ust., in climacteric irregularities of the circulation.

Frequently indicated after: Sil., Sulph.

A single dose often acts curatively for many weeks.

It antidotes mental effects of overuse of tobacco, in patients of sedentary habits who suffer from overmental exertion.

Aggravation

In afternoon or evening; from cold air or dry east wind; sexual excesses; at rest; sultry, moist weather; *before a thunderstorm* (Psor.).

Amelioration

Warmth of bed, hot applications; violent exercise.

Many symptoms, especially those of head, heart and pelvis, are both < and > by rest and exercise.

SILICEA

Pure Silica *Silicic Oxide*

Adapted to the nervous, irritable, sanguine temperament; persons of a psoric diathesis.

Persons of light complexion; fine dry skin; pale face; weakly, with lax muscles.

Constitutions which suffer from deficient nutrition, not because food is lacking in quality or quantity, but from imperfect assimilation (Bar-c., Calc.); oversensitive, physically and mentally.

Scrofulous, rachitic children *with large heads;* **open fontanelles and sutures;** much sweating about the head (lower than Calc.), which must be kept warm by external covering (Sanic.); *distended abdomen;* weak ankles; slow in learning to walk.

Great weariness and debility; wants to lie down.

Nervous debility; exhaustion with erythism; from hard work and close confinement; may be overcome by force of will.

Restless, fidgety, starts at least noise.

Anxious, yielding, fainthearted.

Mental labor very difficult; reading and writing fatigue, cannot bear to think.

Ailments: Caused by suppressed foot-sweat (Cupr., Graph., Psor.); exposing the head or back to any slight draft of air; bad effects of vaccination, especially abscesses and convulsions (Thuj.); chest complaints of stonecutters with total loss of strength.

Want of vital heat, always chilly, even when taking active exercise (Led., Sep.).

Inflammation, swelling and suppuration of glands, cervical, axillary, parotid, mammary, inguinal, sebaceous; malignant, gangrenous.

Has a wonderful control over the suppurative process—soft tissue, periosteum or bone—maturing abscesses when desired or reducing excessive suppuration (affecting chiefly the soft tissues, Calen., Hep.).

Children are obstinate, headstrong, cry when spoken kindly to (Iod.).

SILICEA

Vertigo: Spinal, ascending from back of neck to head; as if one would fall forward, from looking up (Puls.; looking down, Kalm., Spig.).

Chronic sick headache, since some severe disease of youth (Psor.); *ascending from nape of neck to the vertex*, as if coming from the spine and locating in one eye, especially the right (left, Spig.); < draft of air or uncovering the head; > pressure and wrapping up warmly (Mag-m., Stront-c.); > profuse urination.

Constipation: *Always before and during menses* (diarrhea before and during menses, Am-c., Bov.); difficult *as from* **inactivity of rectum;** with great straining, as if rectum was paralyzed; **when partly expelled, recedes again** (Thuj).

Feces remain a long time in the rectum.

Fistula in ano alternates with chest symptoms (Berb., Calc-p.).

Discharge of blood from vagina every time *the child takes the breast* (compare, Crot-t.).

Nipple is drawn in like a funnel (Sars.).

Night walking; gets up while asleep, walks about and lies down again (Kali-br.).

Unhealthy skin; every little injury suppurates (Graph., Hep., Merc., Petr.).

Crippled nails on fingers and toes (Ant-c.).

Takes cold from exposure of feet (Con., Cupr.).

Sweat of hands, toes, feet and axillae; **offensive.**

Intolerable, sour, carrion-like odor of the feet, without perspiration, every evening.

SILICEA

Fistula lachrymalis; ingrowing toe nails (M-arct., Teucr.); panaritium; blood boils; carbuncles; ulcers of all kinds; fistulae, painful, offensive, high spongy edges, proud flesh in them; fissura ani; great pain after stool.

Desire to be magnetized, which > (Phos.).

Promotes expulsion of foreign bodies from the tissue; fish bones, needles, bone splinters.

Relationship

Complementary: Thuja, Sanicula.

Compare: Get., Hep., Hyper., Kali-p., Pic-ac., Ruta, Sanic.

Follows well: After, Calc., Graph., Hep., Nit-ac., Phos.

Is followed well: By, Hep., Fl-ac., Lyc., Sep.

Silicea is the chronic of Pulsatilla.

Aggravation

Cold; during menses, *during new moon; uncovering*, especially the head; *lying down*.

Amelioration

Warmth, especially from wrapping up the head; all the symptoms except gastric, which are > by cold food (Lyc.).

SPIGELIA

Pinkroot   *Loganiaceae*

Adapted to anemic debilitated subjects of rheumatic diathesis; to scrofulous children afflicted with ascarides lumbricoides (Cina, Stann.).

Persons with light hair; pale, thin, bloated, weak; wrinkled, yellow, earthy skin.

Body painfully *sensitive to touch; part touched feels chilly;* touch sends shudder through the whole frame (Kali-c.).

Afraid of sharp, pointed things, pins, needles, etc.

Rheumatic affections of heart (Kalm., Led., Naja); systolic blowing at apex. Aneurysm.

Nervous headache; periodical, beginning in morning at base of brain, spreading over the head and locating in eye, orbit at temple of left side (right side, Sang., Sil.); pain pulsating, violent, throbbing.

Headache; at sunrise, at its height at noon, declines till sunset (Nat-m., Tab.).

Intolerable pressive pain in eyeballs; could not turn the eye without turning the whole body; worse, especially on making a false step.

Sensation: As if eyes were too large for the orbits (Cimic., Com.); *sensitive to touch;* as if a band around head (Cact., Carb-ac., Sulph.).

Copious offensive mucus from posterior nares, drops into throat, causing choking at night (Hydr.).

Sharp, stabbing, sticking pains through eyeballs back into the head; *from cold, damp, rainy weather.*

Prosopalgia: Periodical, left-sided, orbit, eye, malar bone, teeth; *from morning until sunset;* pain tearing, burning, cheek dark red; during *cold, rainy weather;* from tea.

Toothache from *tobacco smoking;* > only on lying down and *while eating* (Plan.); worse from cold air and water; returns from thinking about it.

Scirrhus of sigmoid or rectum, atrocious unbearable pain (Alumn).

Dyspnea: Must lie on right side or with head high (Cact., Spong.); pains in chest are stitching, needle-like.

Chest affections with stitching pains synchronous with pulse, < from motion, < cold, wet weather.

Palpitation: *Violent, visible* and *audible;* from least motion; when bending forward; systolic blowing at apex

Stammering, repeats first syllable three or four times; with abdominal ailments; with helminthiasis.

Relationship

Compare: Acon., Ars., Cact., Dig., Kali-c., Kalm., Naja, Spong., in heart affections.

Aggravation

From motion, noise, touch, turning the eyes; *from every shaking, commotion, or concussion.*

Amelioration

Lying on right side with the head high (Ars., Cact., Spong.).

SPONGIA TOSTA

Roasted Sponge *Spongia*

For the tubercular diathesis.

Especially adapted to diseases of children and women; light hair, lax fibre, fair complexion (Brom.).

Swelling and induration of glands; goitre (Brom.).

Awakens in a fright and feels as if suffocating; as if he had to breathe through a sponge.

Every mental excitement < or increases the cough.

Worse after sleep or sleeps into < (Lach.).

Sore throat, < after eating sweet things.

Thyroid glands swollen even with chin; with suffocative paroxysms at night. Goitre.

Great dryness of mucous membranes of air passages—throat, larynx, trachea, bronchi—"dry as a horn."

Cough: Dry, barking, croupy; rasping, ringing, wheezing, whistling; *everything is perfectly dry, no mucus rale.*

Cough: *Dry, sibilant,* **like a saw** *driven through a pine board;* < *sweets, cold drink;* smoking, *lying with head low,* dry cold winds; < reading, singing, talking, swallowing; > eating or drinking warm things.

Croup: *Anxious, wheezing,* < *during inspiration* (< during expiration, Acon.); < before midnight (< before morning, Hep.).

Palpitation: Violent with pain and gasping respiration; awakened suddenly after midnight with suffocation and great anxiety; valvular insufficiency; before or during menses.

Angina pectoris; contracting pain, heat, faintness, suffocation, anxiety and sweat; < after midnight.

Spermatic cord swollen, painful; testicles swollen, bruised, squeezed; after suppressed gonorrhea or maltreated orchitis.

Relationship

Spongia follows well: After, Acon., Hep., in cough and croup when dryness prevails; after, Spong., Hep., when mucus commences to rattle.

Compare: Arn., Caust., Iod., Lach., Nux-m., sputa loosened but must be swallowed again.

STANNUM

Tin *The Element*

Extreme exhaustion of mind and body.

Sinking, empty, all-gone sensation in stomach (Chel., Phos., Sep.).

Sad, despondent, feels like crying all the time, but crying makes her worse (Nat-m., Puls., Sep.); faint and weak, especially when *going down stairs;* can go up well enough (Borx.—reverse of Calc.).

STANNUM

Headache or neuralgia; pains begin lightly and *increase gradually* to the highest point and then *gradually decline* (Plat.).

Colic: > by hard pressure, or by laying abdomen across knee or shoulder (Coloc.); lumbrici; passes worms.

Menses: Too early, too profuse; sadness before; pain in malar bones, during.

Leucorrhea; great debility weakness seems to proceed from chest (from abdomen, pelvis, Phos., Sep.).

Prolapsus uteri, worse during stool (with diarrhea, Podo.); *so weak she drops into a chair* instead of sitting down.

While dressing in the morning has to sit down several times to rest.

Nausea and vomiting: In the morning; from the odor of cooking food (Ars., Colch.)

When singing or using the voice, aching and weakness in deltoid and arms.

Great weakness in chest; < from talking, laughing, reading aloud, singing; **so weak, unable to talk.**

Cough: Deep, hollow, shattering, strangling; concussive in paroxysms of three coughs (of two, Merc.); dry, while in bed, in evening; *empty sensation in chest*.

Expectoration: Profuse, like the white of an egg; *sweetish, salty* (Kali-i., Sep.); sour, putrid, musty; yellow, green pus (heavy, green, salty, Kali-i.); during the day.

Hoarseness: Deep, husky hollow voice; relieved for the time by coughing or expectorating mucus.

Sweat: Mouldy, musty odor; after 4 a.m. every morning; on neck forehead; very debilitating.

Relationship

Complementary: Pulsatilla.

Stannum follows well: After, Caust., and is followed by Calc., Phos., Sil., Sulph., Tub.

Aggravation

Laughing and singing, talking, *using the voice*; lying on right side; *drinking anything warm* (from cold drinks, Spong.).

Amelioration

Coughing or expectorating relieves hoarseness; hard pressure (Coloc.).

STAPHYSAGRIA

Stavestcre   *Ranunculaceae*

For the mental effects of onanism and sexual excesses.

Very sensitive to slightest mental impressions; least action or harmless word offends (Ign.).

Great indignation about things done by others or by himself; grieves about consequences.

Apathetic, indifferent, low-spirited, weak memory from sexual abuses (Anac., Aur., Nat-m., Ph-ac.).

Ailments from pride, envy or chagrin.

STAPHYSAGRIA 301

Ill-humored children cry for things which, after receiving, they petulantly push or throw away (Kreos.).

Was insulted; being too dignified to fight, subdued his wrath and went home sick, trembling and exhausted (the reverse of Nux-v.).

Sensation of a round ball in forehead sitting firmly there even when shaking the head.

Mechanical injuries from sharp-cutting instruments; *post-surgical operations;* stinging, smarting pains, like the cutting of a knife.

For the bad effects of: Onanism, sexual excesses, loss of vital fluids; chagrin, mortification; unmerited insults; indignation, with vexation or reserved displeasure (Aur.).

Nervous weakness; as if done up after much hard work.

Styes, chalazae on eyelids or upper lids, one after another, *leaving hard nodosities in their wake* (Con., Thuj.).

Toothache: *During menses;* sound as well as decayed teeth; painful *to touch of food or drink,* but not from biting or chewing; < drawing cold air into mouth; < from cold drinks and after eating.

Teeth turn black, show dark streaks through them; cannot be kept clean; crumble; *decay on edges* (at the roots, Mez., Thuj.); scorbutic cachexia.

Craving for tobacco.

Extreme hunger even when stomach is full of food.

Sensation as if stomach and abdomen were hanging down relaxed (Agar., Ip.., Tab.).

STAPHYSAGRIA

Colic: After lithotomy or ovariotomy; attending abdominal section (Bism., Hep.).

Urging to urinate, has to sit at urinal for hours; in young married women; after coition; after difficult labor (Op.); burning in urethra when *not urinating;* urging and pain *after* urinating in prostatic troubles of old men; prolapse of bladder.

Painful sensitiveness or sexual organs, vulva so sensitive can scarcely wear a napkin (Plat.).

Onanism; persistently dwelling on sexual subjects; constantly thinking of sexual pleasures.

Spermatorrhea: With sunken features; *guilty, abashed look;* emission followed by backache, weakness; prostration and relaxation or atrophy of sexual organs.

Cough, only in the daytime, or only after dinner, worse after eating meat; after vexation or indignation; excited by cleaning the teeth.

Croupy cough in winter alternating with sciatica in summer; *cough excited by tobacco smoke* (Spong.).

Backache, < at night in bed, and in the morning before rising.

Arthritic nodosities of joints, especially of the fingers (Caul., Colch., Lyc.); inflammation of phalanges with sweating and suppuration.

Sleepy all day, awake all night; body aches all over.

In fever; ravenous hunger for days before attack.

Eczema: Yellow, acrid moisture oozes from under crusts; new vesicles form from contact of exudation; by scratching one place after itching ceases, but appears in another.

Fig-warts: Dry, pediculated, cauliflower-like; after abuse of mercury (Nit-ac., Sab., Thuj.).

Relationship

Compare: Caust., Coloc., Ign., Lyc., Puls., and Staph. act well after each other; Caust., Coloc., Staph., follow well in order named.

Inimical: Ran-b., either before or after.

Aggravation

Mental affections; from anger, indignation, grief, mortification; loss of fluids; tobacco, onanism; sexual excesses; from the touch on affected parts.

STRAMONIUM

Thorn Apple *Solanaceae*

Adapted to: Ailments of young plethoric persons (Acon., Bell.); especially children in chorea; mania and fever delirium.

Delirium: Loquacious, talks all the time, sings, makes verses, raves; simulates Bell. and Hyos., yet differs in degree.

The delirium is more furious, the mania more acute, while the congestion, though greater than Hyos., is much less than Bell., never approaching a true inflammation.

Disposed to talk continually (Cic., Lach.); incessant and incoherent talking and laughing; **praying, beseeching, entreating;** with suppressed menses.

Desire light and company; cannot *bear to be alone* (Bism.); *worse in the dark and solitude;* cannot walk in a dark room.

Awakens with a shrinking look, as if afraid of the first object seen.

Hallucinations which terrify the patient.

Desire to escape, in delirium (Bell., Bry., Op., Rhus-t.).

Imagines all sorts of things; that she is double, lying crosswise, etc. (Petr.).

Head feels as if scattered about (Bapt.).

Eyes wide open, prominent, brilliant; pupils widely dilated, insensible; contortion of eyes and eyelids.

Pupils dilate when child is reprimanded.

Face hot and red with cold hands and feet; circumscribed redness of cheeks, blood rushes to face; risus sardonicus.

Stammering: Has to exert himself a long time before he can utter a word; makes great effort to speak; distorts the face (Bov., Ign., Spig.).

Vomiting: As soon as *he raises head from pillow;* from a bright light.

Convulsions: With consciousness (Nux-v.; without, Bell., Cic., Hyos., Op.); renewed by sight of bright light, of mirror or water (Bell., Lyss.).

Twitching of single muscles or groups of muscles, especially upper part of body; chorea.

Hydrophobia; fear of water, other excessive aversion to liquids (Bell., Lyss.); spasmodic constriction of throat.

No pain with most complaints; **painlessness** is characteristic (Op.).

Sleepy, but cannot sleep (Bell., Cham., Op.).

Relationship

Stramonium often follows: Bell., Cupr., Hyos., Lyss.

In metrorrhagia from retained placenta with characteristic delirium, Sec. often acts promptly when Stram. has failed (with fever and septic tendency, Pyrog.).

After overaction, from repeated doses of Bell. in whooping cough.

Aggravation

In the dark; when alone; looking at bright or shining objects; after sleep (Apis, Lach., Op., Spong.); when attempting to swallow.

Amelioration

From bright light; from company; warmth.

SULPHUR

Brimstone; Flowers of Sulphur *The Element*

Adapted to persons of a scrofulous diathesis, subject to venous congestion; especially of portal system.

Persons of nervous temperament, quick motioned, quick tempered, plethoric, skin excessively sensitive to atmospheric changes (Hep., Kali-c., Psor.).

For lean, stoop-shouldered persons who walk and sit stooping; walk stooping like old men.

Standing is the worst position for Sulphur patients; they cannot stand; every standing position is uncomfortable.

Dirty, filthy people, prone to skin affections (Psor.).

Aversion to being washed; *always < after a bath.*

Too lazy to rouse himself; too unhappy to live.

Children: *Cannot bear to be washed or bathed* (in cold water, Ant-c.); emaciated, big-bellied; restless, hot, kick off the clothes at night (Hep., Sanic.); have worms, but the best selected remedy fails.

When carefully selected remedies fail to produce a favorable effect, especially in acute diseases, it frequently serves to rouse the reactive powers of the system; clears up the case (in chronic disease, Psor.).

Scrofulous, psoric, chronic diseases that result from suppressed emotions (Caust., Psor.).

Complaints that are continually relapsing (menses, leucorrhea, etc.); patient seems to get almost well when the disease returns again and again.

SULPHUR

Congestion to single parts; eyes, nose, chest, abdomen, ovaries, arms, legs, or any organ of the body marking the onset of tumors or malignant growths, especially at climacteric.

Sensation of burning: On vertex; and smarting in eyes; in face, without redness; of vesicles in mouth; and dryness of throat, first right then left; in stomach; in rectum; in anus, and itching piles, and scalding urine; like fire in ripples (Ars.); in chest, rising to face; of skin of whole body, with hot flushes; in spots, between scapulae (Phos.).

Sick headache every week or every two weeks; prostrating, weakening (Sang.); with hot vertex and cold feet.

Constant heat on vertex; cold feet in daytime with burning soles at night, wants to find a cool place for them (Sang., Sanic.); puts them out of bed to cool them off (Med.); cramps in calves and soles at night.

Hot flushes during the day with weak, faint spells, passing off with a little moisture.

Bright redness of lips as if the blood would burst through (Tub.).

Weak, empty, gone or faint feeling in the stomach about 11 a.m. (10 or 11 a.m. > by eating, Nat-c.); cannot wait for lunch; frequent weak, faint spells during the day (compare, Zinc.).

Diarrhea: After midnight; painless; **driving out of bed early in the morning** (Aloe, Psor.); as if the bowels were too weak to retain their contents.

Constipation: Stools hard, knotty, dry, as if burnt (Bry.); **large, painful,** *child is afraid to have the stool on account of pain,* or pain compels child to desist on first effort; alternating with diarrhea.

The discharge both of urine and feces is *painful to parts over which it passes;* passes large quantities of colorless urine; **parts around anus red, excoriated;** *all the orifices* of the body are *very red;* all discharges acrid, excoriating wherever they touch.

Menses: Too early, profuse, protracted.

Menorrhagia, has not been well since her last miscarriage. "A single dose at new moon."—Lippe.

Boils: Coming in crops in various parts of the body, or a single boil is succeeded by another as soon as first is healed (Tub.).

Skin: Itching, voluptuous; scratching >; "feels good to scratch"; scratching causes burning; < from heat of bed (Merc.); soreness in folds (Lyc.).

Skin affections that have been treated by medicated soaps and washes; hemorrhoids, that have been treated with ointments.

To facilitate absorption of serous or inflammatory exudates in brain, pleura, lungs, joints, when Bryonia, Kalium mur. or the best selected remedy fails.

Chronic alcoholism; dropsy and other ailments of drunkards; "they reform," but are continually relapsing (Psor., Tub.).

Nightly suffocative attacks, wants the doors and windows open; becomes suddenly wide awake at night;

drowsy in afternoon after sunset, wakefulness the whole night.

Happy dreams, wakes up singing.

Everything looks pretty which the patient takes a fancy to; even rags seem beautiful.

Movement in abdomen as of a child (Croc., Thuj.).

Relationship

Complementary: Aloe, Psor.

Ailments from the abuse of metals generally.

Compatible: Calc., Lyc., Puls., Sars., Sep.

Sulph. Calc., Lyc., or Sulph., Sars., and Sep. frequently follow in given order.

Calcarea must not be used before Sulphur.

Sulphur is the chronic of Aconite and follows it well in pneumonia and other acute diseases.

Aggravation

At rest; *when standing; warmth in bed;* washing, bathing; changeable weather (Rhus-t.).

Amelioration

Dry, warm weather; lying on the right side (reverse of Stann.).

SULPHURICUM ACIDUM

Sulphuric Acid H_2SO_4

Adapted to the light-haired, old people, especially women; flushes of heat in climacteric years.

Unwilling to answer questions not from obstinacy, but inaptness.

Feels in a great hurry; everything must be done quickly (Arg-n.).

Pain of gradual and slow-increasing intensity which ceases suddenly when at its height, often repeated (Puls.).

The pain is pressure as of a blunt instrument. Tendency to gangrene following mechanical injuries, especially of old people.

Child has a sour odor despite careful washing (Hep., Mag-c., Rheum).

Sensations as if the brain was loose in forehead and falling from side to side (Bell., Bry., Rhus-t., Spig.).

Aphthe; of mouth, gums, or entire buccal cavity; gums bleed readily; ulcers painful; offensive breath (Borx.)

Chronic heartburn, *sour eructations, sets teeth on edge* (Rob.).

Water drunk causes coldness of the stomach unless mixed with alcoholic liquor.

Sensation as if trembling all over, without real trembling; internal trembling of drunkards.

SULPHURICUM ACIDUM

Bad effects from mechanical injuries, with bruises, chafing and livid skin; prostration (Acet-ac.).

Ecchymosis; cicatries turn blood-red or blue, are painful (turn green, Led.).

Petechia; purpura hemorrhagica; blue spots; livid, red, itching blotches.

Hemorrhage of black blood from all the outlets of the body (Crot-h., Mur-ac., Nit-ac., Ter.).

Concussion of brain from fall or blow where skin is cold and body bathed in cold sweat.

Weak and exhausted from some deep-seated dyscrasia; no other symptoms (Psor., Sulph.).

Relationship

Complementary: Puls.

Compare: Ars., Borx., Calen., Led., Ruta, Rheum, Symph.

In contusion and laceration of soft parts it vies with Calendula.

Follows well: After, Arn., with bruised pain, livid skin and profuse sweat; after, Led. in ecchymosis.

Ailments, from brandy drinking.

Sulphuricum acidum, one part, with three parts of alcohol, 10 to 15 drops, three times daily for three or four weeks, has been successfully used to subdue the craving for liquor. – Hering.

SYMPHYTUM

Comfrey   *Borraginaceae*

Facilitates union of fractured bones (Calc-p.); *lessens peculiar pricking pain;* favors production of callous; when trouble is of nervous origin.

Irritability at point of fracture; periosteal pain after wounds have healed.

Mechanical injuries; blows, bruises, thrusts on the globe of the eye.

Pain in eye after a blow of an obtuse body; snow ball strikes the eye; infant thrusts its fist into its mother's eye (to soft tissues around the eye, Arn.).

Relationship

Compare: Arn., Calen., Calc-p., Fl-ac., Hep., Sil.

Follows well: After Arnica, for *pricking* pain, and soreness of periosteum remaining after an injury.

SYPHILINUM

Syphilitic Virus   *A Nosode*

Pains from darkness to daylight; begin with twilight and end with daylight (Merc., Phyt.).

Pains increase and decrease gradually (Stann.); shifting and require frequent change of position.

All symptoms are worse at night (Merc.); from sundown to sunrise.

Eruptions: Dull, red, copper-colored spots, becoming blue when getting cold.

Extreme emaciation of entire body (Abrot., Iod.).

Heart: Lancinating pains from base to apex, at night (from apex to base, Med.; from base to clavicle, or shoulder, Spig.).

Loss of memory; cannot remember names of books, persons or places; arithmetical calculation difficult.

Sensation: As if going insane, as if about to be paralyzed; of apathy and indifference.

Terrible dread of night on account of mental and physical exhaustion on awakening; it is intolerable, death is preferable.

Fears the terrific suffering from exhaustion on awakening (Lach.).

Leucorrhea: **Profuse,** *soaking through the napkins* and running down to the heels (Alum.).

Headache, neuralgic in character, causing sleeplessness and delirium at night; commencing at 4 p.m.; worse from 10 to 11 and ceasing at daylight (ceases at 11 or 12 p.m., Lyc.); **falling of the hair.**

Acute ophthalmia neonatorum; lids swollen, adhere during sleep; pain intense at night < from 2 to 5 a.m.; pus profuse; > by cold bathing.

Ptosis: Paralysis of superior oblique; sleepy look from drooping lids (Caust., Graph.).

Diplopia, one image seen below the other.

SYPHILINUM

Teeth: Decay at edge of gum and break off; are cupped, edges serrated; dwarfed in size, converge at their tips (Staph.).

Craving alcohol, *in any form.* Hereditary tendency to alcoholism (Asar., Psor., Tub., Sulph., Sul-ac.).

Obstinate constipation for years; rectum seems tied up with strictures; when enema was used the agony of passage was like labor (Lac-c., Tub.).

Fissures in anus and rectum (Thuj.); prolapse of rectum; obstinate cases with a syphilitic history.

Rheumatism of the shoulder joint, or at insertion of deltoid, < from raising arm laterally (Rhus-t.; right shoulder, Sang.; left, Ferr.).

When the best selected remedy fails to relieve or permanently improve, in syphilitic affections.

Syphilitics, or patients who have had chancre treated by local means, and as a result have suffered from throat and skin troubles for years, are nearly always benefited by this remedy at commencement of treatment unless some other remedy is clearly indicated.

Relationship

Compare: Aur., Asaf., Kali-i., Merc., Phyt., in bone diseases and syphilitic affections.

Aggravation

At night, from twilight to daylight.

TABACUM

Tobacco   *Solanaceae*

Diseases originating from cerebral irritation followed by marked irritation of functions of vagi.

Emaciation of cheeks and back.

Complete prostration of entire muscular system.

Sensation of excessive wretchedness.

Icy coldness of surface; *covered with cold sweat.*

Symptoms occur in paroxysms—asthma, sick headache, vertigo, sneezing.

Great despondency with indigestion, palpitation, intermittent pulse.

Vertigo; *death-like pallor,* increasing to loss of consciousness; relieved in open air and by vomiting; on rising or looking backward; **on opening the eyes.**

Sick headache coming on in early morning, intolerable by noon, deathly nausea, violent vomiting; < by noise and light; periodical, lasting one or two days.

Sudden pain on right side of head as if struck by a hammer or a club

Dim-sighted: Sees as through a veil; strabismus, depending upon brain troubles.

Amaurosis, from atrophy of retina or optic nerve.

Face pale, blue, pinched, sunken, collapsed; covered with cold sweat (cold sweat on forehead, Verat.).

Nausea: Incessant, as if seasick; vomiting, on least motion; with faintness; > in open air.

Vomiting: *Violent,* **with cold sweat;** *soon as he begins to move;* during pregnancy, when Lacticum acidum fails (Psor.).

Sea sickness: Deathly nausea, pallor, coldness; < by least motion and > **on deck in fresh, cold air.**

Terrible, faint, sinking feeling at pit of stomach.

Sense of relaxation of stomach with nausea (Ip., Staph.).

Child wants abdomen uncovered, relieves nausea and vomiting; coldness in abdomen (Colch., Elaps, Lach.).

Constipation: Inactive bowel or paralysis of rectum; spasms of sphincter; prolapsus ani; of year's standing; herpes of anus.

Diarrhea: Sudden, yellowish, greenish, slimy; urgent, watery, *with nausea, vomiting, prostration and cold sweat* (Verat.); with extreme faintness; from excessive smoking.

Renal colic: Violent spasmodic pains along ureter, left side (Berb.); deathly nausea and cold perspiration.

Palpitation: Violent when lying on left side; goes off when turning to the right.

Pulse: Quick, full, large; small, intermittent, exceedingly slow; feeble, irregular, almost imperceptible.

Hands icy cold, body warm.

Legs icy cold, from knees down; trembling of limbs.

Relationship

Antidotes, for abuse of tobacco, are:

Ip., for excessive nausea and vomiting.

Ars., for bad effects of tobacco chewing.

Nux-v., for the gastric symptoms next morning after smoking.

Phos., palpitation, tobacco heart, sexual weakness.

Ign., for annoying hicough from tobacco chewing.

Clem. or Plan., **for tobacco toothache.**

Sep., neuralgic affections of right side of face; dyspepsia; chronic nervousness, especially in sedentary occupations.

Lyc., for impotence, spasms, cold sweat from excessive smoking.

Gels., occipital headache and vertigo from excessive use, especially smoking.

Tabacum, potentized (200 or 1000) to relieve terrible craving when discontinuing use.

Amelioration

Open, fresh, cold air; uncovering.

TARAXACUM

Dandelion *Compositae*

For gastric and bilious attacks, especially gastric headaches.

Mapped tongue (Lach., Merc., Nat-m.); covered with a white film with sensation of rawness. This film comes off *in patches*, leaving dark red, tender, *very sensitive spots* (Ran-s.).

Jaundice with enlargement and induration of liver (mapped tongue).

Debility, loss of appetite, *profuse night sweats*, especially when convalescing from bilious or typhoid fever.

Restlessness of limbs in typhoid (Rhus.-t, Zinc.).

Relationship

Compare: Bry., Chel., Hydr., Nux-v., in gastric and bilious affections.

Aggravation

Almost all symptoms appear when sitting; lying down; resting.

TARENTULA

Tarentula: Cuben and Spanish   *Araneideae*

Adapted to highly nervous organisms, especially choreic affections where whole body, or right arm and left leg are affected (left arm and right leg., Agar.).

Constant movement of the legs, arms, trunk, with inability to do anything; twitching and jerking of muscles.

Restlessness, *could not keep quiet in any position;* must keep in motion, *though walking < all symptoms* (reverse of, Rhus-t., Ruta).

Hyperesthesia: Least excitement irritates, followed by languid sadness; extreme, of tips of fingers.

Slight touch along the spine provokes spasmodic pain in chest and cardiac region.

Headache: Intense, as if thousands of needles were pricking in the brain.

Abscesses, boils, felons, affected parts of a *bluish color* (Lach.), and *atrocious burning pain* (Anthraci., Ars.); the *agony of a felon,* compelling patient to walk the floor for nights.

Malignant ulcers; carbuncle, anthrax; gangrene.

Symptoms appear periodically.

Headache, neuralgic < by *noise, touch, strong light,* > by rubbing head against the pillow.

At every menstrual nisus, throat, mouth and tongue intolerably dry, especially when sleeping (Nux-m.).

Sexual excitement extreme even to mania; spasms of uterus; pruritus vulvae becomes intolerable.

Relationship

Similar: To, Apis, Crot-h., Lach., Plat., Myg., Naja, Ther.

Aggravation

Motion; *contact;* **touch of affected parts;** noise; change of weather.

Amelioration

In open air; music; *rubbing affected parts.*

Termini of nerves become so irritated and sensitive that some kind of friction was necessary to obtain relief.

TEREBINTHINIAE

Oil of Turpentine   ***A Volatile Oil***

The urine has the odor of violets.

Tongue: *Smooth, glossy, red,* as if deprived of papillae, or as if glazed (Pyrog.); elevated papillae; coating peels off in patches leaving bright red spots, or entire coating cleans off suddenly (in exanthemata); dry and red; burning in tip (compare, Mur-ac.).

Abdomen extremely sensitive to touch; distention, flatulence, *excessive tympanitis;* meteorism (Colch.).

Diarrhea: Stool, watery, greenish, mucus; *frequent, profuse, fetid, bloody; burning* in anus and rectum *fainting* and *exhaustion,* after (Ars.).

Worms: With foul breath, choking (Cina, Spig.); dry, hacking cough; tickling at anus; ascarides, tapeworm segments passed.

Hematuria: Blood *thoroughly mixed with the urine;* sediment, like coffee-grounds; *cloudy, smoky, albuminous; profuse, dark or black, painless.*

Congestion and inflammation of viscera; kidneys, bladder, lungs, intestines, uterus; with hemorrhage, and malignant tendency.

Purpura hemorrhagica; fresh ecchymosis in great numbers from day to day (Sul-ac.).

Ascites with anasarca in organic lesions of kidneys; dropsy after scarlatina (Apis, Hell., Lach.).

Hemorrhages; *from bowels,* with ulceration; passive, dark with ulceration or epithelial degeneration.

Violent burning and drawing pains in kidney, bladder and urethra (Berb., Cann-s., Canth.).

Violent burning and cutting in bladder; tenesmus; sensitive hypogastrium; cystitis and retention from atony of fundus.

Albuminuria: Acute, in early stages, when blood and albumin abound more than casts and epithelium; after diphtheria, scarlatina, typhoid.

Urine rich in albumin and blood, but few if any casts; < from living in damp dwellings.

Strangury; spasmodic retention of urine.

Relationship

Compare: Alumn., Arn., Ars., Canth., Lach., Nit-ac.

Is recommended as a prophylactic in malarial and African fevers.

THERIDION CURASSAVICUM

Orange Spider   *Araneideae*

Time passes too quickly (too slowly, Arg-n., Cann-i., Nux-m.).

Vertigo: **On closing the eyes** (Lach., Thuj.; on opening them, Tab.; on looking upward, Puls., Sil.); **from any, even least noise;** aural or labyrinthine (Meniere's disease).

Nausea: From least motion, and *especially on closing the eyes;* from fast riding in a carriage.

Headache: When beginning to move; as of a dull heavy pressure behind the eyes; violent, deep, in the brain; < lying down (Lach.); very much < from others walking on the floor, or from least motion of head.

Every sound seems to penetrate through the whole body, causing nausea and vertigo.

Chronic nasal catarrh; discharge thick, yellow, greenish, offensive (Puls., Thuj.).

Toothache; *every shrill sound* penetrates the teeth.

Sea sickness of nervous women; *they close their eyes* to get rid of the motion of the vessel and grow deathly sick.

Violent stitches in upper left chest, below the scapula, extending to neck (Anis., Myrt-c., Pix, Sulph.).

Pains in the bones all over, as if broken.

Great sensitiveness between vertebrae, sits sideways in a chair to avoid pressure against spine (Chinin-s.); < by least noise and jar of foot on floor.

For extreme nervous sensitiveness; of puberty, during pregnancy and climacteric years.

"In rachitis, caries, necrosis, it apparently goes to the root of the evil and destroys the cause." —Dr. Baruch.

Phthisis florida, often effects a cure if given in the easily stages of disease.

In scrofulosis where the best closen remedies fail to relieve.

Relationship

Follows well: After, Calc. and Lyc.

THLASPI BURSA PASTORIS

Shepherd's Purse *Cruciferae*

Profuse passive hemorrhage from every outlet of the body; *blood dark and clotted.*

Metrorrhagia: With violent cramps and uterine colic; in chlorosis; after abortion, labor, miscarriage; at climacteric; with cancer uteri (Phos., Ust.).

Menses: Too early; too profuse; protracted (eight, ten, even fifteen days); tardy in starting, first day merely a show; second day colic, vomiting, a hemorrhage with large clots; each alternate period more profuse.

Hemorrhage or delaying menses from uterine inertia; exhausting, scarcely recovers from one period before another begins.

Leucorrhea: Bloody, dark, offensive; some days before and after menses.

Relationship

Compare: Sinapis, Trillium, Viburnum, Ustilago.

THUJA OCCIDENTALIS

Tree of Life; White Cedar *Coniferae*

Adapted to hydrogenous constitution of Grauvogl, which is related to sycosis as effect is to cause.

Thuja bears the same relation to the sycosis of Hahnemann—fig warts, condylomata and wart-like excrescenses upon mucous and cutaneous surfaces — that Sulphur does to psora or mercury to syphilis.

Acts well in lymphatic temperament, in very fleshy persons, dark complexion, black hair, unhealthy skin.

Ailments from bad effects of vaccination (Ant-t., Sil.); from suppressed or maltreated gonorrhea (Med.).

Fixed ideas: As if a strange person were at his side; as if soul and body were separated; as if a living animal were in abdomen; of being under the influence of a superior power.

Insane women will not be touched or approached.

Vertigo, when *closing the eyes* (Lach., Ther.).

Headache: As if a nail had been driven into parietal bone (Coff., Ign.); or as if a convex button were pressed on the part; < from sexual excesses; overheating; from tea (Sel.); chronic, or sycotic or syphilitic origin.

White scaly dandruff; hair dry and falling out.

Eyes: Ophthalmia neonatorum, sycotic or syphilitic; *large granulations, like warts or blisters;* > by warmth and covering; if uncovered, feels as if a cold stream of air were blowing out through them.

Eyelids: Agglutinated at night; dry, scaly on edges; styes and tarsal tumors; chalazae, thick, hard knots, like small condylomata; after Staphysagria partially > but does not cure.

Ears: Chronic otitis; discharge purulent, like putrid meat; granulations, condylomata; polypi, pale red, cellular, bleeding easily.

Chronic catarrh: After exanthemata; thick, green mucus, blood and pus (Puls.).

THUJA OCCIDENTALIS

Teeth decay at the roots, crowns remain sound (Mez.; on edges, Staph.); crumble, turn yellow (Syph.).

Ranula: Bluish, or varicose veins on tongue or in mouth (Ambr.).

Toothache from tea drinking.

"On blowing the nose a pressing pain in the hollow tooth or at the side of it (Culex)".—Boenninghausen.

Abdomen: As if an animal were crying; motion as if something alive; protrudes here and here and there like the arm of a fetus (Croc., Nux-m., Sulph.).

Distressing, burning pain in left ovarian region when walking or riding, must sit or lie down (Croc., Ust.); worse at each menstrual nisus.

Constipation: Violent pains in rectum compel cessation of effort; *stool recedes, after being partly expelled* (Sanic., Sil.).

Piles swollen, pain *most severe when sitting.*

Diarrhea: Early morning; expelled forcibly with much flatus (Aloe); *gurgling, as water from a bunghole;* < after breakfast, coffee, fat food, vaccination, onions.

Anus fissured, painful to touch, surrounded with flat warts, or moist mucus condylomata.

Coition prevented by extreme sensitiveness of the vagina (Plat.; by dryness, Lyc., Lyss., Nat-m.).

Skin: Looks dirty; brown or brownish-white spots here and there; *warts, large, seedy, pedunculated* (Staph.); eruptions only on covered parts, burn after scratching.

Flesh feels as if beaten, from the bones (Phyt.; as if scraped, Rhus-t.).

Sensation after urinating, as of urine trickling in urethra; severe cutting at *close of urination* (Sars.).

Chill, beginning in the thighs.

Sweat: *Only on uncovered parts;* or all over *except the head* (reverse of Sil.); *when he sleeps, stops when he wakes* (reverse of Samb.); profuse, sour smelling, fetid, at night.

Perspiration, smelling like honey, on the genitals.

When walking the limbs feel as if made of wood.

Sensation as if body, especially the limbs, **were made of glass and would break easily.**

Suppressed gonorrhea: Causing articular rheumatism; prostatitis; sycosis; impotence; condylomata and many constitutional troubles.

Nails: Deformed, brittle (Ant-c.).

Relationship

Complementary: Med., Sab., Sil.

Compare: Cann-s., Canth., Cop., Staph.

Cinnab. is preferable for warts on the prepuce.

Follows well: After, Med., Merc., Nit-ac.

Aggravation

At night; from heat of bed; at 3 a.m. and 3 p.m.; from cold, damp air; narcotics.

TRILLIUM PENDULUM

Wake Robin　　　　　　　　　　　　　　　*Smilaceae*

Hemorrhage: Copious, both active and passive, usually bright red; from nose, lungs, kidneys and uterus (Ip., Mill.).

Tendency to putrescence of fluids.

Epistaxis; profuse, passive, bright red.

Bleeding from cavity after extraction of a tooth (Ham., Kreos.).

Menses: **Profuse, every two weeks, lasting a week or longer** (Calc-p.); after overexertion or too long a ride.

Flooding, with fainting.

Menorrhagia: Flow, *profuse, gushing, bright red; at least movement* (Sab.); from displaced uterus; *at the climacteric; every two weeks*, dark, clotted (Thlas., Ust.).

Hemoptysis: Incipient phthisis, with bloody sputa; in advanced stages with copious, purulent expectoration and troublesome cough.

Sensation as if hips and small of back were falling to pieces; as if sacro-iliac synchondroses were falling apart, wants to be bound tightly; as if bones of pelvis were broken (Aesc.); with hemorrhage.

Profuse uterine hemorrhage at climacteric; flow every two weeks; pale, *faint, dim sight, palpitation, obstruction and noise in ears* (Form.); painful sinking at pit of stomach.

Relationship

Complementary: To Calc-p., in menstrual and hemorrhagic affections.

Compare: Chin., Bell., Kali-c., Mill., Lach., Sep., Sulph., Thlas., Ust.

TUBERCULINUM – BACILLINUM*

Pus (with Bacilli) from Tubercular Abscess   A Nosode

Adapted to persons of light complexion; blue eyes; blonde in preference to burnette; tall, slim, flat, narrow chest; active and precocious mentally, weak physically; the tubercular diathesis.

When with a family history of tubercular affections *the best selected remedy fails to relieve or permanently improve,* without reference to name of disease.

Symptoms ever changing; ailments affecting one organ, then another—the lungs, brain, kidneys, liver, stomach, nervous system—beginning suddenly, ceasing suddenly.

Takes cold easily without knowing how or where; seems to take cold "every time he takes breath of fresh air" (Hep.).

---

* The potencies of Fincke and Swan were prepared from a drop of pus obtained from a pulmonary tubercular abscess or sputa. Those of Heath from a tuberculous lung in which the bacillus tuberculosis had been found microscopically; hence the former was called Tuberculinum and the latter Bacillinum. Both preparations are reliable and effective.

TUBERCULINUM – BACILLINUM

Emaciation rapid and pronounced; losing flesh while eating well (Abrot., Calc., Con., Iod., Nat-m.).

Melancholy, despondent; morose, irritable, fretful, peevish; taciturn, sulky; naturally of a sweet disposition, now on the borderland of insanity.

Everything in the room seemed strange as though in a strange place.

Headache: Chronic, tubercular; pain intense, sharp, cutting, from above right eye to occiput; as of an iron hoop around head (Anac., Sulph.); when the best selected remedy only palliates.

School girl's headache: < by study or even slight mental exertion; when using eyes in close work and glasses fail to >; with a tubercular history.

Acute cerebral or basilar meningitis, with threatened effusion; nocturnal hallucinations; wakes from sleep frightened, screaming; when Apis, Hell., or Sulph., though well selected, fail to improve.

Crops of small boils, intensely painful, successively appear in the nose; *green, fetid pus* (Sec.).

Plica polonica; several bad cases permanently cured after Borx. and Psor. failed.

Diarrhea: Early morning, sudden, imperative (Sulph.); emaciating though eating well (Iod., Nat-m.), stool dark, brown, watery, offensive; discharged with great force; great weakness and profuse night sweats.

Menses: Too early; too profuse; too long-lasting; tardy in starting; with frightful dysmenorrhea; in patients with a tuberculous history.

Tubercular deposit begins in apex of lungs, usually the left (Phos., Sulph., Ther.).

Eczema: Tubercular over entire body; itching intense, < at night when undressing, from bathing; immense quantities of white bran-like scales; oozing behind the ears, in the hair, in folds of skin with rawness and soreness; fiery red skin. Ringworm.

Relationship

Complementary: Psor., Sulph.

When Psor., Sulph., or the best selected remedy fails to relieve or permanently improve; follows Psor. as a constitutional remedy in hay fever, asthma.

Belladonna, for acute attacks, congestive or inflammatory, occurring in tubercular diseases.

Hydrastis to fatten patients cured with Tub.

VALERIANA

Valerian *Valerianaceae*

Excessive nervous excitability; hysterical nervous temperament (Ign., Puls.); persons in whom the intellectual faculties predominate; changeable disposition.

Red parts become white (Ferr.).

Feels light as if floating in the air (Asar., Lac-c.; as if legs where floating, Stict.).

Oversensitiveness of all the senses (Cham., Nux-v.).

Sensation of great coldness in head (on vertex, Sep., Verat.).

Sensation as if a thread were hanging down throat (on tongue, Nat-m., Sil.).

Child vomits: *Curdled milk, in large lumps;* same in stools (Aeth.); *as soon as it was nursed, after mother has been angry.*

Sciatica: Pain < **when standing** *and letting foot rest on floor* (Bell.); when straightening out limb, during rest from previous exertion; > when walking.

Relationship

Compare: Asaf., Asar., Croc., Ign., Lac-c., Spig., Sulph.

For the abuse of Chamomile tea.

For pains in heels: Agar., Caust., Cyc., Led., Mang., Phyt.

VARIOLINUM

Pus from Smallpox Pustule   *A Nosode*

Only fragmentary provings.

Bears the same relation to smallpox that Antitoxin does to diphtheria.

An extended clinical record by competent and reliable observers attests its curative value in variola—

simple, confluent and malignant—as well as in varioloid and varicella.

It has done splendid work in all potencies, from the 6th centessimal to the c.m.

As a preventive of, or protection against, smallpox, it is far superior to crude vaccination and absolutely safe from the sequele, especially septic and tubercular infection. The efficacy of the potency is the stumbling block to the materialist. But is it more difficult to comprehend than the infectious nature of variola, measles or pertussis? Those who have not used it, like those who have not experimentally tested the law of similars, are not competent witnesses. Put it to the test and publish the failures to the world.

VERATRUM ALBUM

White Hellebore　　　　　　　　　　*Melanthaceae*

For children and old people; *the extremes of life;* persons who are habitually cold and deficient in vital reaction; young people of a nervous sanguine temperament.

Adapted to diseases with **rapid sinking of the vital forces; complete prostration; collapse.**

Cold perspiration on the forehead (over entire body, Tab.); with nearly all complaints.

Cannot bear to be left alone; yet persistently refuses to talk.

Thinks she is pregnant or will soon be delivered.

Mania with desire to cut and tear everything, especially clothes (Tarent.); with lewd, lascivious talk, amorous or religious (Hyos., Stram.).

Attacks of fainting from least exertion (Carb-v., Sulph.); excessive weakness.

Sinking feeling during hemorrhage (fainting, Tril.).

Sensation of *a lump of ice on vertex*, with chilliness (Sep.); as of heat and cold at same time on scalp; as if brain were torn to pieces.

Face: **Pale, blue, collapsed; features sunken, hippocratic;** red while lying, becomes pale on rising up (Acon.).

Thirst: Intense, unquenchable, for large quantities of very cold water and acid drinks; wants everything cold.

Craving for *acids or refreshing things* (Ph-ac.).

Icy coldness: Of face, tip of nose, feet, legs, hands, arms, and many other parts.

Cold feeling in abdomen (Colch., Tab.).

Violent vomiting with profuse diarrhea.

Vomiting: Excessive with nausea and great prostration; < by drinking (Ars.); by least motion (Tab.); great weakness after.

Cutting pain in abdomen as from knives.

Cholera: Vomiting and purging; stool, profuse, watery, gushing, prostrating; after fright (Acon.).

Diarrhea: Frequent, greenish, watery, gushing; mixed with flakes; cutting colic, with cramps commencing in hands and feet and spreading all over; prostrating, after fright; < at least movement; with vomiting, cold sweat on forehead during and prostration after (Ars., Tab.).

Constipation: No desire; stool large, hard (Bry., Sulph.); in round, black balls (Chel., Op., Plb.); from inactive rectum; frequent desire felt in epigastrium (Ign.; in rectum, Nux-v.); painful, of infants and children, after Lyc. and Nux-v.

Dysmenorrhea: With vomiting and purging, or exhausting diarrhea with cold sweat (Am-c., Bov.); is so weak can scarcely stand for two days at each menstrual nisus (Alum., Carb-an., Cocc.).

Bad effects of opium eating, tobacco chewing.

Pains in the limbs during wet weather, getting worse from warmth of bed, better by continued walking.

In congestive or pernicious intermittent fever, with extreme coldness, thirst, face cold and collapsed; skin cold and clammy, great prostration; cold sweat on forehead and deathly pallor on face.

Relationship

After: Ars., Arn., Chin., Cupr., Ip.

After Camph. in cholera and cholera morbus.

After Am-c., Carb-v., and Bov., in dysmenorrhea with vomiting and purging.

Aggravation

From least motion; after drinking; before and during menses; during stool; when perspiring; after fright.

Often removes bad effects of excessive use of alcohol and tobacco.

VERATRUM VIRIDE

Green Hellebore   *Melanthaceae*

For full-blooded, plethoric persons.

Congestion, especially **to base of brain,** *chest, spine and stomach.*

Violent pains attending inflammation.

Acute rheumatism, high fever, full, hard, rapid pulse, severe pains in joints and muscles (Bry., Sal-ac.); scanty, red urine.

Child trembles, jerks, threatened with convulsions; continual jerking or nodding of the head.

Nervous or sick headache; congestion from suppressed menses; intense, almost apoplectic, with violent nausea and vomiting.

Congestive apoplexy, hot head, bloodshot eyes, thick speech, *slow full pulse, hard as iron.*

Convulsions: Dim vision; **basilar meningitis;** head retracted; child on verge of spasms.

Cerebro-spinal diseases; with spasms, dilated pupils, tetanic convulsions, opisthotonos; *cold, clammy perspiration.*

Sunstroke, head full, throbbing of arteries, sensitive to sound; double or partial vision (Gels., Glon.).

Tongue: White or yellow with **red streak down the middle;** dry, moist, white or yellow coating, or no coating on either side; feels scalded (Sang.).

Pulse: Suddenly increases and gradually decreases below normal; *slow, soft, weak;* irregular, intermittent (Dig., Tab.).

Veratrum viride should not be given simply to "bring down the pulse", or "control the heart's action," but like any other remedy for the totality of the symptoms.

ZINCUM METALLICUM

Zinc   ***The Element***

Persons suffering from cerebral and nervous exhaustion; **defective vitality;** *brain or nerve power wanting;* too weak to develop exanthemata or menstrual function, to expectorate, to urinate; to comprehend, to memorize.

Incessant and violent fidgety feeling in feet or lower extremities; must move them constantly.

ZINCUM METALLICUM

Always feels better every way *as soon as the menses begin to flow; it relieves all her sufferings;* but they return again soon after the flow ceases.

In the cerebral affections: In impending paralysis of brain; where the vis medicatrix nature is too weak to develop exanthemata (Cupr., Sulph., Tub.); symptoms of effusion into ventricles.

Child repeats everything said to it.

Child cries out during sleep; whole body jerks during sleep; wakes frightened, starts, *rolls the head from side to side;* face alternately pale and red.

Convulsions: During dentition, **with pale face, no heat,** except perhaps in occiput, no increase in temperature (reverse of Bell.); rolling the eyes; gnashing the teeth.

Automatic motion of hands and head, or one hand and head (Apoc., Bry., Hell.).

Chorea: From suppressed eruption; from fright.

Hunger: Ravenous about 11 or 12 a.m. (Sulph.); *great greediness when eating;* cannot eat fast enough (incipient brain disease in children).

Excessive nervous moving of feet in bed for hours after retiring, even when asleep.

Feet sweaty and sore about toes; fetid, suppressed foot-sweat; nery nervous.

Chilblains, painful, < from rubbing.

Spinal affections; *burning along whole length of spine;* backache, *much < from sitting,* > by walking about (Cob., Puls., Rhus-t.).

ZINCUM METALLICUM

Spinal irritation; great prostration of strength.

Cannot bear back to be touched (Chinin-s., Tarent., Ther.).

Can *only void* urine while sitting bent backwards.

Twitching and jerking of single muscles (Agar., Ign.)

Weakness and trembling of extremities; of hands while writing; during menses.

During sweat cannot tolerate any covering.

Relationship

Compare: Hell., Tub., in incipient brain diseases from suppressed eruptions.

Aggravation

Of many symptoms from drinking wine, even a small quantity (Alum., Con.).

Amelioration

Symptoms: Of chest, by expectorating; of bladder, by urinating; of back, by emissions (< by Cob.); general, by menstrual flow.

Is followed well by, Ign. but not by Nux-v., which disagrees.

Inimical: Cham. and Nux-v., should not be used before or after.

THE MATERIA MEDICA
OF
SOME MORE IMPORTANT REMEDIES

ADRENALINUM (Sarcode)
Extract of Suprarenal Bodies $C_3H_3A_2O_1$

Mind
- Despondent and nervous; lack of interest in anything; no ambition; disinclination for mental work; absence of "grit."
- Aversion to mental work, cannot concentrate thoughts.

Head
- Hot headache in left side, extending to right, < by reading and in morning, with a feeling as though the eyes were strained.
- Frontal headache, supraorbital, with congested nose and eyes.
- Burning heat in head, feeling as though he wanted to open eyes wide
- Headache extending all over head but < on left side and over eyes across forehead.
- Severe pain > by pressure on the eyes.
- Headache extending to the ears. All headaches are < in the afternoon or evening; in the evening they

appear about 7 p.m. and last until relieved by a walk in the open air or sleep.
- If headache appears in the afternoon the time is 3 p.m.; always > by walk in the open air, and somewhat relieved by eating and sleeping, but not so completely as by walk in the open air.
- Neuralgic headache; pains start from base of brain, go forward over the head to front and sides; pains are first shooting and seem to be just under the scalp, appear at 11 a.m. and last until 3 or 4 p.m. and disappear by eating, in open air, < in close, warm room.
- Dull aching in the eyeballs with headache, > by pressure and by rubbing the eyes.
- Headache coming on at 11 a.m., lasting until 12:30 at night, > by eating.
- Dull feeling in the head from 3 to 6 p.m.

Eyes
- Strained feeling, congested, feeling as though he wanted to open them wide or press upon them.
- Pain in the right eye. Pressure on the eyes and opening them wide > the headache
- Aching in eyeballs, > by pressure and rubbing.

Ears
- Aching in the left ear accompanies the headache; sharp pain in both ears at times.
- Itching and tickling in right ear, > by boring into ear with finger.

Nose

- On going out into the cold air had a copious watery nasal discharge, < on right side; when indoors, the nose feels full and stopped up.
- Slight stuffiness in the nose, with full feeling at the root of the nose.

Face

- Feels flushed but is not red.
- Flushes of heat over face and head; flushed throughout evening.

Mouth

- Bad taste on waking.
- Tongue coated white, red edge and tip.

Throat

- Vocal cords inflamed; laryngeal catarrh, profuse secretion from the pharyngeal glands of whitish gelatinous mucus which was difficult to loosen.

Stomach

- Appetite increased.
- Sensation of nausea as if he would vomit.
- Nausea before meals, though appetite is good when he once began to eat.
- Appetite increased; ravenous hunger.

Stool

- Loose, brown, semi-solid, passed quickly, with fetid odor.

- Sudden spluttering diarrhea; all over in a minute, followed with burning in anus

Urine
- Strong odor, hot and scalding; frequent, profuse, pale.
- Burning before and during micturition.
- Crystals of sodium oxalate increased while sodium urate appeared during the proving, and was very prominent, no casts.
- Hematuria with severe pain in the renal region; cured.
- Urine more frequent than usual.
- Sexual desire increased, without erections.
- Erections; lascivious dreams all night causing waking from sleep.
- Emissions in early morning without any bad effects.

Respiratory
- Cough from irritation in suprasternal fossa.
- Increase of respiratory movements, soon followed by suffocation and death from paralysis of medulla and pneumogastric (crude drugs).

Back
- Pain especially on the left side; better by sitting up straight or lying straight.

Extremities
- Slight rheumatic pains coming and going down leg.
- Arms and legs go to sleep easily; numbness and tingling from below upwards.

- Corns on the toes.
- Rheumatic pains in left elbow and little finger on waking.
- Legs tired and ache, especially in the calves and below the knees.
- Ankles feel weak and tired
- Painful swelling on first finger of right hand, resulting in a felon.
- Tired aching in arms and legs on walking.

Tissues
- Prolonged contraction of the general muscular system. Repeated injections cause atheroma and heart lesions in animals.
- The skin becomes bronzed; great loss of strength; rapid emaciation; exceedingly rapid pulse; irregular intermitting heart beats; general marked anemia.

Sleep
- Great sleepiness and drowsiness.
- Dullness and sleepiness from 3 to 6 p.m.

BACILLINUM

A Maceration of a Typical Tuberculous Lung

Mind
- Taciturn, sulky, snappish, fretty, irritable, morose, depressed and melancholic even to insanity.

- Fretful ailing, whines and complains; mind given to be frightened particularly by dogs.

Head

- Severe headache, deep in, recurring from time to time, compelling quiet fixedness; < shaking head.
- Terrible pain in head as if he had a tight hoop of iron around it; trembling of hands; sensation of damp clothes on spine; absolute sleeplessness.
- Alopecia areata.

Eyes

- Eczematous condition of eyelids.

Face

- Indolent, angry pimples on left cheek, breaking out from time to time and persisting for many weeks.

Teeth

- Grinds teeth in sleep.
- Imperfectly developed teeth.

Stomach

- Windy dyspepsia, with pinching pains under ribs of right side in mammary line.

Abdomen

- Fever, emaciation, abdominal pains and discomfort, restless at night, glands of both groins enlarged and indurated; cries out in sleep; strawberry tongue.
- Tabes mesenterica; talks in sleep; grinds teeth; appetite poor; hands blue; indurated and palpable glands everywhere; drum belly; spleen region bulging out.

- Inguinal glands indurated and visible; excessive sweats, chronic diarrhea.

Stool and Anus
- Obstinate constipation.
- Passes much ill-smelling flatus.
- Stitch-like pain through piles.

Urinary Organs
- Increased quantity of urine, pale, with white sediment.
- Has to rise several times in night to urinate.

Respiratory System
- Hard cough, shaking patient, more during sleep, but did not waken him.
- Single cough on rising from bed in morning.
- Cough waking him at night; easy expectoration.
- Sharp pain in precordial region arresting breathing.
- Very sharp pain in left scapula, < lying down in bed at night, > by warmth.

Neck and Back
- Glands of neck enlarged and tender.

Lower Limbs
- Tubercular inflammation of knee.

Generalities
- Great weakness, did not want to be disturbed.

Sleep
- Drowsy during day; restless at night; many dreams.

Fever
- Flush of heat (soon after the dose), some perspiration, severe headache deep in.

CHOLESTERINUM
Cholesterine $C_{26}H_{44}O$

Swan appears to have taken his hint from Burnett's work and potentized the remedy, using a gall-stone for his preparations. Like many of the rest of the nosodes originally introduced by Swan, the work was necessarily empirical, yet he affirms after much experience that it is "almost a specific for gall-stone colic; relieves the distress at once." And this after failure with Nux-v., China, Carduus, Podophyllum and other apparently well-selected remedies.

Yingling reports some cures of gall-stone colic and other diseases of the liver in the *Medical Advance*, page 549, August, 1908.

Clarke says, it is found in the blood, in the brain, the yolk of eggs, seeds and buds of plants, but is most abundant in the bile and biliary calculi. It occurs in the form of crystals with a mother-of - pearl luster, and is fatty to the touch. It is soluble in both alcohol and ether.

Ameke claimed to have derived great advantage from its use in cases diagnosed as cancer of the liver, or in such obstinate engorgements that malignancy was suspected.

Burnett claims to have twice cured cancer of the liver with it, and "in hepatic engorgements that by reason of their intractable and slow yielding to well-selected remedies make one think interrogationally of cancer." In such conditions where the diagnosis is in doubt, especially if the patient has been subjected to repeated attacks of biliary colic, Cholesterinum, he claims, is very satisfactory and at times its action even striking.

Yingling reports the following cases:

1st Case:
- Attacks come suddenly and cease suddenly.
- Pain is pushing in region of gall duct.
- Marked acidity of stomach since last attack.
- No appetite; food nauseates.
- Region of liver sore, sensitive to touch or jar, < lying on the sides.

2nd Case
- Vomits bile and becomes very yellow.
- Liver very sensitive and sore; pressure in front or behind very painful, worse in region of gall duct.
- Bending or any sudden motion aggravates.
- Cholesterinum 2m. not only promptly relieved acute attacks, but has effected a practical cure."

ELECTRICITAS
(Atmospheric and Static)

Caspari and his colleagues obtained the symptoms caused by Electricity, natural and artificial, and was first published in *Hom. Bibliot.* Later it appears in Jahr and has recently been republished, with additions by Clarke. Every medical man knows the extreme susceptibility of some persons to the electric fluid and the sufferings they experience on the approach of, and during, a thunderstorm, or the contact of an electric current.

The potencies are prepared from milk sugar which has been saturated with the current.

Characteristics

- Intense nervous anxiety; timid, fearful, sighing; screams through nervous fear; paroxysms of weeping.

- Dreads the approach of a thunderstorm; suffers mental torture before and during an electric storm.

- Heaviness and paralysis of limbs and entire body, feels as if she weighted a ton.

- Electricity should not be used nor electro-thermal baths taken when suffering from a cold, especially if the chest be involved; fatal results have followed.

Relations

- Antidote: Morphinum aceticum, especially the potency. Clarke says: "I have found Phosphorus the best antidote to the effects of storms."

- Compare: The X-ray, Psor., Tub., to remove the susceptibility.

ELECTRICITY

Mind
- Weeping, timid, fearful; sighing; crying out through nervous fear.
- Paroxysms of oppressive anxiety.
- Dread at the approach of a thunderstorm; fear; internal anguish, especially of chest; nervous agitation.
- Involuntary hysterical laughter. Rage. Ill-humor. Unable to comprehend time. Comprehension slow and difficult. Suffers mental torture before and during an electric storm.
- Loss of memory.

Sensorium
- Loss of consciousness.
- Loss of sensibility.
- Dullness of head.
- Stupefaction. Giddiness, especially on stooping.

Head
- Headache; pressure in the forehead, from above downwards, as from a stone.

- Tearing from the nape of the neck to the forehead.
- Painful spasms in the head.
- Sore pain in the occiput.
- Disagreeable shocks, generally in the occiput.
- Roaring in the whole sinciput.

Outer Head
- Feeling of coldness on the vertex.
- The growth of the hair is considerably promoted.

Eyes
- Sensation as if the eyes were deep in the head.
- Sensation as if something would come out of the eyeball.
- Inflammation of the eyes; profuse lachrymation.
- Dim-sightedness.
- Blindness.
- Black point before the right eye.
- Everything looks yellow.

Ears
- Darting in the right ear, from the throat.
- Drawing from the jaws into the ears.
- Swelling of the inner ear.
- Blisters behind the ears full of an acrid fluid.
- Whizzing in the ears, or sensation as if obstructed by a plug.

Nose
- Loss of smell.
- Discharge of a milky fluid from the nose.

Face
- Expression of terror in the countenance.
- Scurf in the face, on the arms and body.
- Large blisters on the cheeks.

Teeth
- Tearing in the upper teeth, proceeding from the head.
- Pain as from subcutaneous, ulceration in old sockets of the molar teeth.

Mouth and Pharynx
- Increased secretion of saliva.
- Foam at the mouth.
- The tongue is very sensitive, particularly at the tip.
- Swelling of the tongue.

Throat
- Loss of speech, inability to articulate.
- Blisters on the palate, the epidermis becoming detached.
- Constant titillation in the throat.
- Inflammation of the pharynx.

Stomach, Nausea and Vomiting
- Heartburn.
- Ptyalism.

- Nausea, also after a meal.
- Desire to vomit.
- Vomiting with sore throat.
- Hematemesis.

Stomach
- Sense of repletion in the stomach, after a slight meal.

Abdomen
- Cutting in the abdomen at the approach of a thunderstorm.

Stool
- Black-yellow, liquid stools, having a fetid smell.
- Drawing up of the testes during stool.
- Violent pressing in the anus (during menses).
- Burning at the anus.
- Flowing hemorrhoids.

Urinary Organs
- Frequent micturition.
- Incontinence of urine.
- Discharge of blood with the urine.

Female Sexual Organs
- Appearance of the menses (while in the electric bath).
- Black and thick menstrual blood.
- Profuse menses, with pressing in rectum.
- Leucorrhea, first thin, then thick, with coagula of the size of a hazel nut.

Larynx and Trachea
- Cough with violent titillation in the throat and pressure in the forehead from within outward.

Respiration
- Asthma all one's life, with palpitation of the heart and disposition to faint.

Chest
- Palpitation of the heart, with fever, or with headache or with oppressive anxiety and bright red face.
- Chest and arms become stiff, almost paralyzed; unable to walk.
- Heaviness and stiffness of chest and shoulders, felt like marble.

Back
- Boils in the back and nape of the neck.
- Stinging in a swollen cervical gland.

Upper Limbs
- Frightful pains in the arms and lower limbs.
- Paralysis of the arms.
- Trembling of the hands.
- Swelling of the hand, also red or sudden.
- Feeling of numbness in the tips of the fingers.
- Blister filled with a greenish, sanguinous fluid on the finger which discharges the bottle.

Lower Limbs
- Burning in the foot, up to the knees, particularly at night.

- Coldness of the lower extremities up to the abdomen, in summer, during a cool wind.
- Tingling in the soles of the feet. Sensation as of a broad ring around the malleoli.
- Intense suffering of electric shocks through left foot and entire left side of body to head, repeated at every discharge during a thunderstorm.

Sleep
- Yawning, with shuddering over the whole body.
- Sleeplessness for two months.

Fever
- Shuddering over the body, every morning with yawning.
- Chilliness, then dry, short heat.
- Frequent alternation of chilliness and heat, with sore throat.
- Chilliness with profuse sweat, with painful spasms in the head and along the back.
- Excessive night sweat in an arthritic individual, without relief; sweat with anxiety during a thunderstorm.

Skin
- Violent pains and swelling of the foot which had been frozen twelve years ago.
- Red pimples on the spot touched by the sparks.
- White vesicles.
- The skin becomes blackish.

- Ecchymosis.

General symptoms
- Pains in the limbs.
- Drawing through all the limbs, extending to the tips of the fingers and toes.
- Shock through the whole body, proceeding from the malar bone.
- Tingling in the electrified parts.
- Violent burning of the parts which are in contact with the chain.
- General languor after a meal.
- Relaxation of the nerves and muscles.
- Fainting.
- Stiffness of the limbs.
- Paralysis of single limbs, particularly the lower.
- Trembling of the limbs particularly of those which have received the shock.
- Subsultus tendinum.
- Painful spasms along the back from below upward.
- St. Vitus' dance.
- Aggravation of epileptic fits.
- Intense suffering with paralysis of nervous and muscular system.
- Heavy sensation as if she weighed a ton.

LAC FELINUM

Cat's Milk

Mind

- Great depression of spirits.
- Very cross to every one.
- Fear of falling downstairs, but without vertigo.
- Mental illusion that the corners of furniture, or any pointed object near her, were about to run into eyes; the symptom is purely mental; the objects do not appear to her sight to be too close (asthenopia).

Head

- Dull pain in forehead in region of eyebrows.
- Actual pains on vertex.
- Actual pain over left eye and temple.
- Pain in head < from reading.
- Pain in forehead, occiput, and left side of head, with rigidity of cords of neck (splenius and trapezius), and heat in vertex; the pain in forehead is heavy, pressing down over eyes (headache).
- Intense pain from head along lower jaw, causing mouth to fill with saliva.
- Crawling on top of brain (asthenopia).
- Weight on vertex (asthenopia).
- Terrible headache penetrating left eyeball to centre of brain, with pain in left supraorbital region extending through brain to vertex (headache).

LAC FELINUM

- Burning on left temple near eye, < at night (keratitis).

Eyes

- Sharp lancinating pain through centre of left eyeball leaving it very sore internally, and causing profuse lachrymation (from the 1 m.).
- Heavy pressure downwards of eyebrows and eyelids, as if the parts were lead.
- Inclination to keep eyes shut.

    (Have had great success with it in eye cass, especially where there is severe pain in back of orbit, indicating choroiditis — Swan).

- On looking fixedly, reading, or writing, darting pain from eyes nearly to occiput; much < in right eye (asthenopia).
- When reading, letters run together, with dull aching pain behind eyes, or shooting in eyes, the confused sight and shooting being < in right eye; symptoms excited by catching cold or by over-fatigue (asthenopia).
- Pain in eyes, back into head, extremely sharp, with a sensation as if eyes extended back; great photophobia to natural or artificial light; any continued glare results in this pain (improved).
- Photophobia.
- Stye on left upper lid.
- Eyes get bad every September.
- Eyes ache by gaslight.

- A black spot before right eye. Moving with the eye when in sunlight.
- Sensation of sand in right eye on waking.

Teeth
- Pain in all the teeth as the hot pain from head touched them.

Mouth
- Sensation as if tongue were scalded by a hot drink.
- Redness under tongue, on gums, and whole buccal cavity.
- Loss of taste.
- Brassy taste in mouth.
- Salivation, tongue enlarged and serrated at edges by teeth.
- Very sore mouth.

Throat
- Tough mucus in pharynx.
- Stringy, tough mucus in pharynx, cannot hawk it up and has to swallow it; when it can be expectorated it is yellow.
- Posterior wall of pharynx slightly inflamed, with sensation of soreness.

Stomach
- No appetite.
- Great desire to eat paper.
- Stomach sore all around just below the belt, < left side.

- Heat in epigastrium.
- Great soreness and sensitiveness of epigastric regions.

Abdomen
- Pain in abdomen and back, as if menses are about commencing.
- Great weight and bearing-down in pelvis, like falling of the womb, as if she could not walk; < when standing.
- Pain in pelvis through hips on pressure, as when placing arms akimbo.

Stool and Rectum
- Natural stool, but very slow in passing, at 2 a.m.
- Stool long, tenacious, slipping back when ceasing to strain; seeming inability of rectum to expel its contents.

Urinary Organs
- Frequent desire to urinate, urine very pale.

  (Obstruction in urinating, has to wait).

Female Sexual Organs
- Leucorrhea ceased on third day and reappeared on fourth day.
- Furious itching of vulva, inside and out; yellow leucorrhea. (Dragging pain in left ovary).

Respiratory Organs
- Dryness of rim of glottis.

Chest
- Very much oppressed for breath, continuing for several days; it is a difficulty in drawing a long breath, or rather that requires the drawing of a long inspiration, for it seems as if the breathing was done by upper part of lungs alone.

Upper Limbs
- Pain in right side of left wrist when using index finger.

Lower Limbs
- Left foot feels cold when touched by right foot. Legs ache.

Sleep
- Dullness, sleepiness, gaping.
- Heavy, profound sleep, not easily awakened.

Fever
- Cold and heat alternately, each continuing but a short time.

Generalities
- Entire right side from crown to sole felt terribly weak, heavy, and distressed, so that it was difficult to walk. (Constant nervous trembling, especially of hands, as in drunkards).

LAC VACCINUM

Cow's Milk

Mind
- General nervousness, with depression of spirits, feeling as though about to hear bad news.
- Mental confusion, lasting a long time after proving.
- Mental prostration, came on so suddenly, was unable to collect her thoughts or write her thoughts or write her symptoms.

Head
- Vertigo: Falls backwards if she closes her eyes.
- Fullness of head as it too large and heavy.
- Vertigo.

Eyes
- Dull pain over right eye, and very slight dull feeling over left eye.
- Eyes have a blur, or dimness, or obscurity of sight, off and on for a few moments at a time.

Ears
- Ears felt stopped up; felt deaf in both ears, although she could hear as before.

Mouth
- Had a dirty, yellow-coated tongue, which felt parched.
- Sour taste.
- Acid saliva staining handkerchief yellow.

- Ulcers on tongue, flat, white, sunken; tongue swollen, exceedingly sensitive, covered with white, slimy mucus on the parts not ulcerated; breath extremely fetid; sores extend to inside cheeks and tonsils; deglutition painful.

Throat
- Sensation of plug in throat or larynx.

Appetite
- Thirst for cold water in quantities; drank three tumblerfuls during evening.

Stomch
- Had a swelling or bloating of stomach (3d d).
- At 10:30 a.m. sour taste, nausea, but no rising or vomiting (1 h).
- Eructations.

Abdomen
- Pain proceeding from sternum, extending across abdomen about an inch below umbilicus.
- Constant intolerable flatulence, begins an hour after drinking milk for lunch and lasts all the afternoon.
- Borborygmus, with loud, noisy rumbling (200).

Stool
- Obstinate constipation; stool hard, dry; in impacted balls; can be passed only with great straining.
- Passage of stinking flatus, in large quantity, which relieves.

Female Sexual Organs
- White watery leucorrhea; pain in sacrum.
- Drinking a glass of milk will promptly suppress the flow until next menstrual period.
- Menses, suppressed, delayed by putting hands in cold water.
- "Nausea of pregnancy with desire for food > by drinking milk."

Back
- Sensation of plug in throat or larynx.

Respiratory Organs
- Pains in sacrum.

Lower Limbs
- Piercing or lancinating pain in each hip joint, not severe.
- Short rheumatic pains in knee and tarsal joints when walking.

Skin
- Brown crusts, having a greasy appearance, especially in corners of mouth, similar to what are called "butter-sores."

Generalities
- The pains in chest, abdomen, hips, thighs, and knees were all felt on right and left sides simultaneously.

MAGNETIS POLI AMBO

The Magnet

Mind and Disposition

- While attending to his business in the daytime, he talks aloud to himself, without being aware of it.
- Excessive exhaustion of the body, with feeling of heat, and cool sweat in the face with unceasing and, as it were, hurried and over-strained activity.
- Hurried headlessness and forgetfulness; he says and does something different from what he intends, omitting letters, syllables and words.
- He endeavors to do things, and actually does thing contrary to his own intentions.
- Wavering irresolutions, hurriedness.
- He is unable to fix his attention on one object.
- The things around him strike him like one who is half dreaming.
- He inclines to be angry and vehement; and after he has become angry, his head aches as if sore.
- He is disposed to feel vexed; this gives him pain, especially a headache, as if a nail were forced into his head.

Sensorium

- Vertigo in the evening after lying down, as if he would fall, or resembling a sudden jerk through the head.

- When walking he staggers from time to time, without feeling giddy.
- The objects of sight seem to be wavering, this makes him stagger when walking.

Head

- Whizzing in the whole head, occasioned by the imposition of magnetic surfaces on the thighs, legs and chest.
- The head feels confused as when one takes opium.
- When endeavoring to think of something and fatiguing his memory, he is attacked with headache.
- Headache, as is felt after catching cold.
- Headache occasioned by the least chagrin, as if a sharp pressure were made on a small spot in the brain.
- Pain in the region of the vertex, at a small spot in the brain, as if a blunt nail were pressed into the brain; the spot feels sore to the touch.
- Sensation on top of the head, as if the head and whole body were pressed down.

Face

- Cold hands, with heat in the face and smarting sensation in the skin of the face.
- Intolerable burning prickings in the muscles of the face, in the evening.
- Sweat in the face without heat, early in the morning.

Eyes

- Dilated pupils with cheerfulness of the mind and body.
- Fiery sparks before the eyes, like shooting stars.
- Sensation in the eye as if the pendulum of a clock were moving in it.
- White, luminous, sudden vibrations, like reflections of light, at twilight, on one side of the visual ray, all round.
- Itching of the eyelids and eyeballs in the inner canthus.
- Sensation as if the eyelids were dry.
- Twitching of the lower eyelid.

Ears

- Fine whistling in the ear, coming and going like the pulse.
- Whizzing before the ears.
- Electric shocks in the ear.
- Hard hearing without noise in the ear.

Nose

- Illusion of smell: Smell of manure before the nose, from time to time he imagines he has a smell before the nose such as usually comes out of a chest full of clothes which had been closed for a long while.

Teeth and Jaws

- Metallic taste on one side of the tongue.
- Tearing pain in the periosteum of the upper jaw,

coming with a jerk and extending as far as the orbit; the pain consists in a tearing, boring, pricking and burning.
- Darting-tearing pain in the facial bones, especially the antrum Highmorianum, in the evening.
- When taking a cold drink, the coldness rushes into the teeth.
- Looseness of the teeth.
- Toothache, excited by stooping.
- The gums of a hollow tooth are swollen and painful to the touch.
- Aching pain of the hollow, carious, teeth.
- Uniform pain in the roots of the lower incisors, as if the teeth were bruised, sore or corroded.

Mouth and Pharynx
- Shocks in the jaws.
- Shock in the teeth with burning.
- Pain of the submaxillary gland as if swollen, early in the morning in open air.
- Ptyalism every evening with swollen lips.
- Bad smell from the mouth which he does not perceive himself also with much mucus in the throat.
- Continual fetid odor from the mouth, without himself perceiving it, as in incipient mercurial ptyalism.
- Burning of the tongue, and pain of the same when eating.

Taste and Appetite
- Hunger, especially in the evening.
- He has an appetite, but the food has no taste.
- He has a desire for tobacco, milk, beer, and he relishes those things; but he feels satisfied immediately after commencing eating.
- Aversion to tobacco, although he relished it.
- Want of appetite without any loathing, repletion or bad smell.

Stomach
- Eructations, tasting and smelling like the dust of sawed or turned horn.
- The eructations taste of the ingesta, but as if spoiled.
- Crackling and cracking in the pit of the stomach, as when a clock is wound up.
- Sensation of an agreeable distension in the region of the diaphragm.
- Pressure in the epigastrium, as from a stone, especially when reflecting much.
- Tensive aching and anxious repletion in the epigastrium.

Abdomen
- The flatulence moves about in the abdomen, with loud rumbling, painless incarceration of flatulence in various small places of the abdomen, causing a sharp aching pain and an audible grunting.
- Loud, although painless rumbling, especially in the

lesser intestines, extending under the pubic bones and into the groin, as if diarrhea would come on.

- Emission of short and broken flatulence, with loud noise and pains in the anus.
- Loud rumbling in the abdomen, early in the morning when in bed; afterwards colic as if from incarceration of flatulence.
- Putrid fermentation in the bowels, the flatulence has a fetid smell and is very hot.
- Qualmish sensation and painfulness in the intestines, as if one had taken a resinous cathartic or rhubarb, with painful emission of hot, putrid flatulence.
- Every emission of flatulence is preceded by pinching in the abdomen.
- Tensive and burning pain in the epigastrium and hypogastrium, followed by a drawing and tensive pain in the calves.
- Itching of the umbilicus.

Stool
- Diarrhea without colic.
- Constipation as if the rectum were constricted and contracted.
- Violent hemorrhoidal pain in the anus after stool, erosive as if sore, and as if the rectum were constricted.
- Burning at the anus when sitting, as in hemorrhoids.
- Itching hemorrhoids.

- Blind harmorrhoids after soft stool, as if the varices on the margin of the anus felt sore, both when sitting and walking.
- Prolapsus recti when going to stool

Urinary Organs
- Burning in the bladder, especially in the region of the neck of the bladder, a few minutes after urinating.

Male Genital Organs
- Burning in the urethra, in the region of the caput gallinaginis, during an emission of semen.
- Early in the morning he feels a burning in the region of the vesiculae seminales.
- Nightly emissions of semen.
- Violent continuous erections, early in the morning when in bed, without any sexual desire.
- Want of sexual desire, aversion to an embrace.
- The penis remains in a relaxed condition, in spite of all sexual excitement.
- The prepuce retreats entirely behind the glans.
- Swelling of the epididymis, with simple pain when feeling it or during motion.
- Itching smarting of the inner surface of the prepuce.

Female Genital Organs
- Menses had caused a few days before, returned next day after imposing the magnetic surface and continued ten days.

Larynx

- Frequent fits of nightly cough which does not wake him.
- Convulsive cough.
- Mucus in the trachea which is easily hawked up, evening and morning.
- Violent fit of cough, with profuse expectoration of blood.

Chest and Lungs

- Asthma after midnight when waking and reflecting, occasioned by mucus in the chest, diminished by coughing.
- Spasmodic cough, with shocks in the chest and anxious breathing, and visible oppression of the chest.
- Violent oppression of the chest, tearing in the stomach and bowels, and beating in the shoulders.

Back

- Painful stiffness of the cervical vertebra in the morning, during motion.
- Crackling in the cervical vertebra in the morning during motion.
- Pain in the omo-hyoid muscle, as if it would be attached with cramp.
- Pain in the back when standing or sitting quiet.
- Burning in the dorsal spine.
- Twitching of the muscles of the back and sensation as if something were alive in them.

- Pain in sacro-lumbar articulation, in the morning when in bed lying on the side, and in daytime when stooping a long time.
- Shock or jerk in the small of the back, almost arresting the breathing.

Upper Limbs
- Tearing jerkings in the muscles of the arm when staying in a cold place.
- Shocks in the top of the shoulder which caused the arms to recede from the body with a jerk.
- Shocks in the arm joints and head, as if those parts were beaten with a light and small hammer.
- Prickings in the arms.
- Beating and throbbing in all the joints of the arms and fingers.
- Deep-seated pain in the arm, extending as far as the elbow, the arm going to sleep and trembling spasmodically.
- Drawing from the head down to the tip of the fingers.
- The hands are icy cold the whole day, for several days, from touching the centre of the bar.
- Pain in the wrist joint, as if a tendon had become strained, or as if an electric shock were passing through the parts.

Lower Limbs
- Attacks of cramp in the calves and toes after walking.
- Drawing from the hips to the feet, leaving a burning along that tract.

- Violent shocks of the right lower limb, occasioned by a burning emanation from the chin and neck through the right side.
- Fiery burning in the upper and lower limbs; when the right limb touched the left one, if seemed as if the latter were set on the fire by the former.
- Pain in the upper part of the tarsal joints, as if the shoe had pinched him, and as if a corn were there.

Sleep
- Coma vigil early in the morning for several hours; after sunrise, sopor or deep sleep set in full of heavy, passionate dreams, for instance, vexing dreams; the sopor terminates in a headache as if the brain were sore all over, disappearing after rising.
- Lascivious dreams, even during the siesta, with discharge of the prostatic fluid.

Skin
- The recent wound commences to bleed again.
- The wound, which is almost healed, commences to pain again like a recent wound.
- Boils break out on various parts of the body, passing off soon.
- Corrosive pain in various parts, for example, below the ankle.

General Symptoms
- Dull, numb pain.
- Jerking shock, causing the trunk to bend violently upward and forward as low down as the hips, with cries.

- Fits of fainting, palpitation of the heart and suffocation.
- Long-lasting swoons, in which she retained her consciousness.

MAGNETIS POLUS ARCTICUS
North Pole of the Magnet

Mind and Disposition
- Out of humor and weary.
- Weeping mood with chilliness and a disposition to feel chilly.
- Sadness, in the evening; he made to weep, contrary to his will, after which his eyes felt sore.
- Indolent fancy; he sometimes felt as if he had no fancy at all.
- Indolent mind.
- While attending to his business, he talks aloud to himself.
- He makes mistakes easily in writing.
- Hasty, bold, quick, firm.
- Calm, composed mood, devoid of care.

Sensorium
- (Vertigo, sensation as if she would fall in every direction.)
- Vertiginous motion in one side of the head.

- Sensation of intoxication, like a humming in the head.
- Dullness of the head with desire for open air.
- Weak memory, but he feels cheerful.

Head
- Headache, consisting in a sore and bruised pain in the surface of the brain, in the sinciput and in one of the temples.
- Sensation as if the head were pressed down by a load.
- Disagreeable, compressive sensation in the head, and as if one part of the brain were pressed in.
- Headache, as if the temples were pressed asunder.
- Violent headache the whole afternoon, as if the brain were pressed asunder.
- Rush of blood to the head, and suffusion of heat in the cheeks.
- Drawing-boring pain in the right temple, accompanied with a spasmodic pain below the right malar bone.
- Aching pain over the left temporal region, externally.
- Pushing tearing in the head behind the left ear when sitting.

Eyes
- Cold movement as of a cold breath in the eyes.
- The eyes protrude.
- Staring look.

- Itching in the inner canthus and in the margin of the eyelids.
- Painful feeling of dryness in the eyelids in the morning on waking.
- Jerking and drawing in the eyelids.
- Drawing in the eyelids with lachrymation.
- Pricking in the eyelids.
- Lachrymation early in the morning.
- Excessive lachrymation; the light of the sun is intolerable.
- Burning in the weak right eye; it became red and filled with water (the magnet being held in contact with the weak right eye for a quarter of an hour).
- Coldness in the weak eye for three or four minutes (the magnet being held in contact with that eye for two minutes).
- Uneasy motion of the eye, with a good deal of water accumulating in either eye.
- Sensation as of a cobweb in front of the eyes.
- Formication between the two eyes.
- Strong drawing over the eye, in the surface of the cheek, ear, extending into the upper maxillary bone (the magnet being in contact with the eye).

Ears

- Fine ringing in the opposite ear (immediately).
- Whizzing a drawing sensation in the ear.
- Ringing in the ear of same side.

- A kind of deafness, as if a pellicle had been drawn over the right ear, after which heat is felt in the ear.

Nose
- Illusion of smell: He imagines the room smelled of fresh whitewash and dust, he imagines the room smells of rotten eggs, or of the contents of a privy.
- Violent bleeding at the nose, for three afternoons in succession, increasing every afternoon, and preceded by an aching pain in the forehead.
- Redness and heat of the tip of the nose, followed by hot, red circumscribed spots on the cheeks.

Face
- Intensely painful tightness in the face, extending as far as the tonsils.
- Drawing in the left cheek.

Jaws and Teeth
- Drawing-aching pain coming from the temple, below the mastoid process, between the sterno-cleido-mastoideus muscle and the ramus of the lower jaw.
- Toothache as if the tooth would be torn out, worse after a meal, and when sitting or lying down, improving when walking.
- Toothache in the direction of the eye, a very quick succession of pecking in the hollow tooth, with swollen inflamed gums and a burning cheek; the toothache increased very much immediately after a meal, improved when walking in the open air, but aggravated in a smoky room.

- Throbbing in the hollow tooth (immediately), followed by a pressure in the tooth as if something had got into the tooth, with drawing in the temples.
- Throbbing in the tooth, with burning in the gums, and swollen, hot cheeks, with burning pain and heat in the cheeks, in the afternoon.
- The toothache ceases when walking in the open air, and returns in the room.
- Aching in the hollow teeth, with swelling of one side of the face.
- Toothache with jerks through the periosteum of the jaw, the pain being a darting-aching, digging-tearing, or burning-stinging pain.
- The toothache is worse after eating and in the warm room.
- Numbness and insensibility of the gums of the painful tooth.
- Drawing pain in the hollow tooth, and fore teeth, increased by anything warm; with redness of the cheek during the pain.
- Swelling of the gums of a hollow tooth, painful when touched with the tongue.
- Toothache, as if the gums were sore or cut, increased by the air entering the mouth.

Mouth

- Sore pain in the left corner of the mouth, when moving it, as if an ulcer would form.
- Painful humming in the hollow teeth of the lower

jaw, worse on the right side, the toothache ceases during eating.

Appetite and Taste
- Sourish taste in the morning, as if one were fasting.
- Greedy appetite at supper.

Stomach
- Frequent eructation of mere air.
- Drawing in the pit of the stomach, extending into the right chest.

Abdomen
- Spasmodic contractive sensation in the hypogastrium, externally and internally, early in the morning.
- Flatulent colic immediately after supper; sharp pressure in every part of the abdomen from within outward, as if the abdomen would burst; relieved when sitting perfectly still.
- Flatulent colic early in the morning, immediately after waking; the flatulence was pressed upward towards the hypochondriac region, with tensive pains in the whole abdomen, causing a hard pressure here and there, accompanied with a qualmishness and nausea which proceeded from the abdomen, and was felt both in motion and when at rest.
- Gurgling in the abdomen as if a quantity of flatulence were incarcerated, causing a writhing sensation, which rises up to the pit of the stomach, and causes eructations.

- Relaxed condition of the abdominal ring, increasing from day to day; hernia threatens to protrude, especially when coughing.
- Sore pain in the abdominal ring, when walking.
- Boring pain above the left abdominal ring, from within outward, as if hernia would protrude.
- Inguinal hernia.

Stool
- Drawing, almost dysenteric pain in the hypogastrium, early in the morning, followed by difficult expulsion of the very thick feces.
- Stinging-pinching in the rectum.

Genital Organs
- Nightly involuntary emission.

Respiratory Organs
- Dry cough causing a painful rawness in the chest, especially in the night after getting warm in bed, having been chilly first.
- Racking and spasmodic cough while falling asleep, hindering sleep.
- Suffocative, spasmodic cough about midnight.

Chest
- Pressure in the region of the heart (immediately).
- When walking in the open air he imagines that heat is entering chest, passing through the pharynx.

Back
- Crackling or cracking in the cervical vertebrae especially in the atlas, during motion.

- Pain as if bruised in the middle of the spine, when bending the spine backward.
- Gurgling and creeping sensation between the scapule.
- Twitching in the posterior lumbar muscles.
- Pain as if bruised in the left shoulder joint both during motion and rest, painless when touching it.

Upper Extremities
- Cramp-like sensation in the arm, and as if it had gone to sleep.
- Violent coldness in the arm over which the magnet had been moved (in a female in magnetic sleep, after being touched with the north pole magnet).
- Prickling pain in the arm as far as the shoulder, especially in the long bones of the forearm.
- Sore pain in the right shoulder when walking in the open air.
- Stiffness and rigidity in the right tarsal and carpal joints, at night when in bed.
- Painful and almost burning itching in dorsum of the middle phalanx of the little finger, as if the part had been frozen; the place was painful to the touch.

Lower Extremities
- Tearing with pressure in the outer side of the knees down to the outer ankle.
- Excessive weakness of the lower limbs, when walking as if they would break.

- Rigid tension in the hamstrings when rising from a seat, as if too short.
- Sore pressure in the corns, which had been painless heretofore, when pressing the feet ever so little.
- Sudden lancinations in the heels, big toe and calf when sitting.
- Painful crawling in the toes of the right foot.

Sleep

- Constant drowsiness in the daytime.
- Lascivious dreams the whole night.
- She saw a person in a dream, and next day she saw that person in reality for the first time.
- Restless sleep; he tosses about and his bed feels too warm.

Fever

- Sensation of coldness or coolness over the whole body as if she were dressed too lightly, or as if she had taken cold, without shuddering; immediately after she had a small loose stool which was succeeded by pressing.
- Shuddering all over at the moment when the north pole was touched by the tip of the tongue.
- Cool sweat all over.
- Heat in one of the cheeks, accompanied with a feeling of internal heat, irritable disposition and talkativeness.

MAGNETIS POLUS ARCTICUS

Skin
- Crawling over the skin.

General Symptoms
- Continuous digging-up stitches in various parts, becoming sharper and more painful, in proportion as they penetrate more deeply into the flesh.
- Tensive sensation in the adjoining parts.
- Bruised pain in the adjoining parts, and as if one had carried a heavy burden.
- Tremulousness through the whole body, especially in the feet.
- Tremor in the part touched by the magnet (immediately).
- Nervousness with trembling, uneasiness in the limbs, great distension of the abdomen, anxiety, solitude and great nervous weakness.
- Sensation of coldness in the part which was touched by the magnet.
- Drawing in the periosteum of all the bones, as is felt at the commencement of an intermittent fever (but without chilliness of heat).
- The faintness, the bruised and painful sensation in the limbs was worse in the open air.

MAGNETIS POLUS AUSTRALIS
South Pole of the Magnet

Mind and Disposition
- Want of cheerfulness; he is low spirited, as if he were alone, or as if he had experienced some sad event, for three hours.
- Weeping immediately.
- Despondency (the first hours).
- Great discouragement, dissatisfaction with himself.
- Want of disposition to work and vexed mood.
- Taciturn, he is not disposed to talk.
- He wants to be alone, company is disagreeable to him.
- Violent anger excited by a slight cause; he becomes trembling and hurried, and uses violent language.
- Wild, vehement, rude, both in language and action (he does not perceive it himself); he asserts with violence, reviling others with distorted countenance.
- Great quickness of fancy.

Sensorium
- Unsteadiness of the mind; he is unable to fix his ideas; things seem to flit to and fro before his senses; his opinions and resolutions are wavering, which occasions a kind of anxious and uneasy condition of the mind.
- Vertigo as if intoxicated, as if he were obliged to stagger, some vertigo even while sitting.

Head

- Rush of blood to the head, without heat.
- Heaviness of the head, with a sort of creeping or fine digging in the head.
- Fine crawling in the brain as of a number of insects, accompanied with heaviness of the head.
- Drawing-tearing pain in the left brain, resembling a slow, burning stitch.
- Pressure in the occiput, in alternate places.
- Headache in the occiput, most violent in the room, but disappearing in the open air (in the first hours).
- Spasmodic contractive headache in the region between the eyebrows.
- The skin on the forehead feels as if dried fast to the skull.

Face

- Sensation in the face (and in the rest of the body) as if cold air were blowing upon it.

Eyes

- Watery eyes from time to time.
- Painful, smarting dryness of the eyelids, especially perceptible when moving them, mostly in the evening and morning.
- Deficient sight: Things looked dim, also double, when touching the nape of the neck.

Ears

- Tearing pains in the cartilages of the outer and inner ear, extending very nearly as far as the inner cavities.

- Roaring in the ears, which he felt more in the upper part of the head.
- Noise in the ears, like the motion of a wing.
- Sensation as of the whizzing of the wind in the ears, early in the morning; he feels it as far as the forehead.
- Inflammation of the outer ear, the grooves of that portion of the ear assuming the appearance of some rhagades.
- Occasional stitches and ringing in the ear.

Jaws and Teeth
- Toothache, aggravated by warm drink.
- Tearing - jerking in the upper jaw towards the eye, in the evening.
- Dull pain with intensely painful stitches in hollow teeth.

Mouth
- Sensation of swelling in the tongue, and heat in the organs of speech.

Throat
- Burning in the pharynx, a sort of strangulation from below upwards, with a feeling of heat.

Appetite and Taste
- Indifference to milk, bordering on aversion, early in the morning.

Nausea and Vomiting
- Inclination to vomit, early in the morning after waking.

- Fits of nausea when stooping forward, apparently in the stomach.

Abdomen

- Loud rumbling in the abdomen.
- Flatulent colic at night; portions of flatulence seem to spring from one place to another, which is painful, and causes disagreeable grumbling sensation, or a sore pinching pressure from within outward in many places, depriving him of sleep, short flatus goes off now and then with pain, but affords no relief.
- Drawing pain in the right side of the abdomen, scarcely permitting him to walk.
- Tearing colic occasioned by (reading?) and walking, and appeared by sitting, especially in the epigastrium (early in the morning).
- Distended abdomen in the evening immediately before going to bed, with colicky pains.
- Emission of quantity of flatulence.
- Sensation as if the abdominal ring were enlarged, and as if hernia protruded; every turn of the cough causes a painful dilation of the ring.

Stool

- Frequent desire for stool, causing nausea, but she is unable to accomplish anything.
- Continual contraction and constriction of the rectum and anus, permitting scarcely the least flatulence to be emitted.

Urinary Organs
- Relaxation of the sphincter vesicae (immediately).
- Incontinence of urine.
- Smarting pain in the forepart of the urethra, during the emission of urine, as if the urine were acrid or sour.

Male Sexual Organs
- Drawing in the spermatic cord, early in the morning with the testicle hanging down, as if pulled or distended; the testicle is even painful to the touch.
- Jerking in the spermatic cord.
- Slow, fine, painful drawing in the spermatic cord.
- Tearing in the spermatic cord.
- Spasmodic drawing up of the testi s, in the night.
- Pain in the penis, as if several fleshy fibres were torn or pulled backwards.
- Red spot, like a pimple, on the corona glandis and on the internal surface of the prepuce, without sensation.
- The glans is red and inflamed, with itching and tension.
- Nocturnal emission (in a person affected with hemiplegia); it had not taken place for years past. (Note by *Hahnemann*—After this emission the paralysis became worse; the sick limb seemed dead to him).
- Impotence: Embrace with the proper sensations and erection; but at the moment when the semen is about

to be emitted, the voluptuous sensation is suddenly arrested, the semen is not emitted; and the penis becomes relaxed.

Female Sexual Organs
- The menses, which had already lasted the usual time, continue to flow for six days longer, only during motion, not when at rest; every discharge of blood is accompanied with a cutting pain in the abdomen. (Note by *Hahnemann*—This woman held the south pole, touching at the same time the middle of the bar. The south pole appears to excite hemorrhage and especially from the uterus, as its primary effect; the north pole seems to act in the contrary manner.)
- The menses, which were to appear in a few days, appeared four hours after the south pole had been touched, but the blood was light-colored and watery.

Respiratory System
- Shortness of breath in the pit of the stomach.

Chest
- Palpitation of the heart.

Back
- Gnawing and smarting in the back.

Upper Limbs
- Crawling in the left arm, from above downward, resembling small snakes.
- Quick, painful jerking, in the arms, from above downward.
- Jerking in the fingers which are touched by the magnet.

- Sense of heat and jerking in the finger touching the magnet.
- Beating in the finger in contact with magnet.

Lower Extremities
- Drawing, with pressure, in the muscles of the thighs, worse during motion.
- Sense of coldness in the right thigh.
- Drawing pain in the outer side of the bend of the knee.
- Tearing with pressure in the patella (worse during motion), and aggravated by feeling the part.
- Cracking of the knee joint during motion.
- Itching-burning, slow stitch in the side of the calf.
- Soreness of the inner side of the nail of the big toe in the flesh, as if the nail had grown into the flesh on one side; very painful, even when slightly touched.
- Pinching occasioned by the shoes on top and on the sides of the toes, and near the nail of the big toe when walking, as from corns.

Sleep
- Frequent yawning (with chilliness).
- Sleepless and wakeful before midnight, and no disposition to go to sleep.
- Restless, frequently turns from side to side, in the night when in bed.
- Dreams about fires.
- He quarrels and fights in a dream.

- Unusual beating in the region of the heart.

Fever
- Chills in the room the whole day, especially after an evening nap.
- Chilliness of the legs upto the knee, with a sensation of heat and blood to the heat.
- Feeling of coldness all over, in the evening (without shuddering), without thirst (except at the commencement of the chilliness), and without being actually cold; at the same time he feels out of humor, everything was disagreeable to him, even the meal, two hours after he was covered with heat and sweat all over, without thirst.
- During the chilliness, or the feeling of coldness, he was quite warm, but he was obliged to lie down, and to cover himself well; his mouth was very dry; afterwards he was covered with a profuse sweat all over, without feeling hot; on the contrary, he felt a constant shuddering over the perspiring parts, as if they were covered with goose-skin; accompanied with a sensation as of a breeze blowing into the ears.
- Warmth all over, especially in the back.

Skin
- Corrosive itching in the evening, when in bed, on the back and other parts of the body.
- Itching, stinging, tearing, here or there, in the evening, when in bed.

General Symptoms

- Bruised pain in all the limbs, so that he imagined he was lying on stones, on whatsoever side of the body he lay.
- Stiffness of the joints.
- Lightness of the whole body.
- Laziness and heaviness of the whole body, accompanied with a feeling of anxiety, as if he were threatened with paralysis, and as if he would fall, accompanied with a feeling of heat in the face and the whole body, mingled with shuddering.

MALANDRINUM

The Grease of Horses

Mind

- Confusion and lassitude of the mental faculties with a dread of any mental exertion and a lack concentration, an entirely new and unusual experience which continued several weeks after stopping the remedy.
- Comprehension difficult.
- Memory weakened and impaired; great difficulty in remembering what was read.
- Sharp darting pain first in left temple then in right. Confusion and lassitude of the mental faculties; lack of concentration and a dread of any mental exertion.
- Melancholy with general fatigue.

Head External

- Pustular eruption on scalp. Sensation of weariness at junction of atlas with cranium, every morning on rising.
- Itching on scalp, especially in the evening.
- Excessive oily dandruff (an entirely new experience) the fourth week after pustules dried up.
- Impetigo covering head from crown to neck and extending behind ears.
- Thick, greenish crusts with pale, reddish scabs, itching in the evening.
- Impetigo, covering back of head, extending over back to buttocks, labia and even into vagina.

Head

- Front and occipital headache, backache, weariness and chilliness, lasting one day.
- Frontal headache, no appetite, bilious vomiting and weariness.
- Dizziness.
- Frontal headache, dizziness, backache.
- Temporal headache, dizziness, backache.
- Terrible headache, bone pains, vomiting (bilious), chilliness, diarrhea, malaise.
- Heaviness in the head.
- Headache and backache, stiffness of neck, loss of appetite, constipation, and great weariness (following vaccination).
- Eruption on forehead, crusty with intense itching.

Face
- Eczema facialis; intense burning, much edema, oozing viscid fluid.
- A yellowish honeycomb crust on upper lip.

Ears
- Profuse purulent, greenish-yellow discharge, mixed with blood.

Mouth
- Tongue, coated yellow; with red streak through middle, cracked and ulcerating down middle; swollen.
- Horribly offensive breath.
- Canker on left border of tongue, which spreads in all directions; tongue sore, unable to speak.
- In one case in which I was using Malandrinum 30 as a prophylactic of variola, it cured a very stubborn case of aphthe.— H.S. Taylor.

Throat
- Sore and swollen < left side. Left tonsil swollen; yellow ulcer with clear-cut, well-defined edges persistent for several days; rough scraping sensation like a corn husk or a foreign body, which must be removed mechanically, painless swallowing.
- Left tonsil swollen and inflamed.
- Throat symptoms and pains in throat begin on left side, and extend to right.
- Ulcerated sore throat and tendency to extend downward, invading the larynx.

Appetite; Throat
- Thirstless; water nauseates.

Teeth and Gums
- Gums swollen, ulcerated, receding from teeth; bleed easily when touched; unable to brush the teeth from sore and bleeding gums.
- A dark, brown, tenacious mucus mixed with blood and pus exudes from ulcerated gums.
- Sordes on the teeth.

Stomach
- Nausea after eating; vomiting of bilious matter.
- Empty, faint, "all gone" sensation, with faintness and trembling, not > by eating, though desire for food is very marked.

Abdomen
- Pains around umbilicus.

Stool
- Diarrhea: Yellow, bloody, slimy; very changeable, worse in the morning; acrid, excoriating; child had a dried-up mummified appearance; sleepless and has not nursed for 24 hours.
- Dark, thin, cadaverous-smelling stool.
- Diarrhea; acrid, yellow, offensive, followed by burning in anus and rectum.
- Dark brown, foul-smelling, almost involuntary diarrhea; pains in abdomen.
- Dark brown, painless diarrhea.

- Black, foul-smelling diarrhea; weariness, nausea, dizziness.
- Yellow, foul-smelling, almost involuntary diarrhea and great weariness.
- Black, foul-smelling, diarrhea, malaise and weariness.
- Bowels inactive, no desire; move after enema, but leave sore bruised sensation in rectum for hours; dreads stool.

Urine
- Great sensitiveness of bladder on waking; bladder irritable, frequent desire to urinate.

Male Sexual Organs
(Child constantly handles the penis).

Female Sexual Organs
- Vagina closed with thick impetiginous crusts; yellowish, greenish, brown in color.

Back
- Intense pain across small of back.
- Pain along back as if beaten.
- Backache was intense in the sacral region; in the dorsal region under the shoulder blades, chiefly the left side; it was almost unbearable (Dr. B. from three doses of the 200th).

Upper Limbs
- Impetiginous crusts on extensor sides of forearms. Rhagades in palms and fingers.

Lower Limbs
- Petechia on both thighs < on left.
- Knock-knee.
- Weak ankles, easily turn on making a false step.
- Profuse foot-sweat with carrion-like odor; toes so sore unable to walk; only > was when feet were bared and elevated.
- Soles of feet bathed in sweat, scald and burn when covered or warm.
- Large blisters on soles of both feet—no change of shoes—skin exfoliated on both feet.
- Feet "go to sleep" upon least provocation, a sensation never before observed.
- Deep rhagades, sore and bleeding, on soles of feet > in cold weather and after bathing.
- Sore in all limbs and joints.
- "Run arounds" on all nails of hands and feet.

Skin
- Eczema of face and scalp, with burning, stinging, itching.
- Impetigo on extensors of forearms.
- Dry, rough, unhealthy skin remaining for years after vaccination.
- Skin rough, dry, harsh.
- Palms and soles thick; deep rhagades < in cold weather, < from washing with any kind of soap.
- Skin greasy; oily eruption, and hair excessively oily.

- Pustules slow to develop but never ending; as one healed another appeared.
- Eruption in hollow of arms and knees, red scaly with intense itching < when becoming warm.

Sleep
- Restless sleep; dreams of trouble, of quarrels.
- For the bad effects of vaccination has been used with best results.
- When used as a prophylactic for variola has proved protective in many cases, and also prevented vaccination from "taking".
- Lower half of body affected; greasy skin; greasy eruption. Slow pustulation, never ending, as one healed another appeared.—Burnett.
- Bad effects of vaccinations; has cured cases of unhealthy, dry, rough skin, remaining for years after vaccination in small pox, measles and impetigo.—Clarke.
- Eczema facialis; oozing of a viscid fluid; intense burning, much edema; small scales, exfoliated < from bathing at night; > in cold air.—Thompson.
- Impetigo covering back of head, extending over whole back to buttocks and even into vagina, covering labia and extensors of forearms.
- Boils. Malignant pustules.
- *Bad effects of vaccination.*
- Small dusky red spots on legs, not disappearing on pressure.

MALARIA OFFICINALIS

Mind
- Feels stupid and sleepy.
  (Very thoughtful).

Head
- Feeling as though he would become dizzy
- Waving dizziness on falling asleep.
- Dizziness on rising from reclining position.
- Dull aching through forehead and temples.
  (Dull headache, dizzy and drowsy).
- Frequent attacks of headache, especially in the forehead.
- Throbbing pain all over head.
- Vertigo; confused sensation; worse by walking, turning around, rising or stooping.
- Headache beginning in forehead, extending all over head.

Eyes
- Aching above inner angle of right eye.
- Eyes feel heavy and sleepy.
  (Eyes weak, blurring; reading difficult).
- Eyes burn like coals of fire.

Ears
- Drawing pain in right external ear.

Nose
- A kind of concentration of feeling at root of nose and just above, as though I should have a severe cold like hay-fever.

Face
- Itching on right cheek over malar bone (and various parts of face and limbs); > by slight rubbing or scratching.
- Face becomes warm as if flushed; and spreads over body.

Mouth
- Pain in upper left teeth.
- Sensation on point of tongue as if a few specks of pepper were there.
- Saliva more profuse than usual, keeps him swallowing often.
- Tongue coated slightly yellowish-white.
  (Bitter taste, parched mouth; tongue white.)
- Tongue white, with brown streak down the middle.
- Tongue while and thickly coated.
- Mouth very dry, subjectively, but really moist.

Appetite
- Wants cold drinks.
- Can't eat anything; vomits everything.
- Craves sour.
- Thirsty; craves cold water.

- No appetite; aversion to food, thought of it sicken.
- Thirsty for lemonade; not so much for water.
- Variable; craves potatoes, apples, beefsteak.
- Bitter, nauseating, bad taste in the mouth.
- Dryness at root of tongue; buccal cavity seems constricted and contracted.

Stomach
- Unusually hearty appetite (for supper).
- Odor from cooking is pleasing, but no desire for dinner; on sitting down eats a good dinner with relish.
- Feels better after eating dinner.
- Easy belching, several times, no taste.
- Qualmish.
- Nausea.
- Retching and gagging from hawking mucus.

Abdomen
- Sense of heat in abdomen.
- Uneasiness in lower abdomen.
- Liver, spleen and kidneys affected.

    (Cannot breathe on account of pain in liver, < lying down, > hard pressure).
- (Drawing or pricking in liver).

    (Cramping in liver, pain under right scapula).
- Great uneasiness through abdomen, sense of heaviness.

- Constipation.
- Diarrhea, no pain; weakness in bowels.
- Steady, dull pains in region of liver > after urinating.
- Aching under right scapula; cramp with soreness and sensitiveness in region of liver; from pressure < by lying down.

Stool and Anus
- Diarrhea.
- Diarrhea in morning, stools thin, yellow, foul.

Respiratory Organs
- Shallow breathing, which seems from languor, desire to breathe occasionally.
- Residence in malarial districts is said to cure phthisis.
- A consumptive constitution is protected against malaria.

Chest
- Tired feeling through chest and abdomen.
- Constant hacking cough, half minute guns, when talking and turning over in bed.
- Frequent sighing, takes a deep inspiration; restless and nervous.

Neck and Back
- Neck feels tired, with slight aching in upper parts on moving the head.
- Lumbar region tired as though it would ache.

(Rheumatism of back and limbs, with lameness).

- Stiff neck, and right arm and shoulders painful and helpless.

  (Aching under right scapula; cramping in liver).
- Backache in lumbar region, shoots up back; worse when first lying down; worse after walking; better lying on the abdomen.

Upper Limbs
- A sense of coldness ascending over body from the legs. Gout.
- Limbs get numb and cold.
- Aching in both elbows.
- Aching and tired feeling in wrists; tired ache in the hands.
- Arms tired.
- Hands seem to be semi-paralyzed, useless, but can use them by force of will.
- Very cold hands during the day; hands and feet very cold at night.

Lower Limbs
- Pain, upper part of right ilium.
- Tired ache in knees and for some distance above and below.
- Aching in an old (cured) bunion on left foot.
- Legs restless, feel like stretching and moving them.
- Soles of the feet cold, almost numb.
- Right knee weak and painful, worse when bending, and raising up.

Generalities

- General sense of weariness; from a very short walk; especially through pelvis, sacral region, and upper thighs; strong desire to lie down.
- A kind of simmering all through the body.
- Typhoidal, semi-paralytic condition (No. III).
- Rheumatism.
- Rheumatic paralysis and emaciation.
- Feels very weak and languid; restless; does not want to move.
- Great weakness as though he had a long illness, with loss of appetite.
- Great exhaustion.
- Must have doors and windows open; a close room < head and stomach, and fresh, cool air chills her.

Skin

(Skin, eyes, and face very yellow).

- Skin dry all over; no sweat at all.

Sleep

- Impelled to lie down, and on falling asleep a sense of waving dizziness passes all over, preventing sleep.
- Gaping, yawning, and desire to stretch.
- Sleep all the time; can go to sleep while standing.
- Sleepy and drowsy, but sleep does not relieve; wakes up weary and unrefreshed.

Fever
- Coldness ascending over body from legs.
- A feeling as if he would have a chill, then as if he would become feverish, though neither is very marked.
- Intermittent; quotidian; tertian (No. II).

  (Ague every other day, weak and drowsy between attacks).

  (Dumb chills).
- Shooting pains all over in the muscles; bones ache.
- High fever during night; also in the morning.
- Chill begins about noon; every other day. Icy cold from hips down; chilly all over; fever worse about the trunk, and slight general sweat.
- Aching all over body, especially in arms and legs; chilly sensation, then breaks out in slight perspiration; frequent recurring attacks.
- Chilly every second day followed by heat; profuse sweat during the night; wakes up chilly and takes cold as perspiration ceases.

Stool
- Hemorrhoids for many years; external bleeding; no pain but very unpleasant.
- Diarrhea; four of five motions daily of thin, bloody, streaked mucus; no fecal matter.

Limbs in General
- Sensation of fatigue in upper extremities first; later extending to lower extremities and entire system.

- Dull pain in the muscles of the back, lumbar region; uneasy; tired.
- Dull aching pain in left sciatic nerve, and on outer surface of left hip.
- Sensation of burning flush, rising from knees to throat, but without sweat; relieved by lying down.
- Dull pain in right hip with soreness and tenderness on pressure in the sheaths of the muscles about the hip and tendons of muscles of the thigh.
- Waking at midnight, feet extremely hot with burning palms and soles; this was followed by profuse sweat on lower part of body, more marked on flexor surfaces and on the back.
- Drawing, shooting pain on left hypochondrium, extending down left leg.
- Arms feel heavy.
- Burning of hands and feet; aching of hands and arms.

Nerves
- Great restlessness all night, worse towards morning. Could not find a position in which he could rest.

Hypochondria
- Dull throbbing pain in hepatic region for three days, relieved by pressure of corset and by lying on the painful side.

THYROIDINUM

Thyroid Extract   *A Sarcode*

Trituration of the fresh thyroid gland of sheep or calf. Attenuation of a liquid extract of the gland.

Mind

- Depression.
- Fretfulness and moroseness gave way to cheerfulness and animation.
- Delirium of persecution (three cases observed, one fatal, the result of taking Thyr. in tablets to reduce obesity).
- Sudden acute mania occurring in myxedema, perfectly restored mentally and bodily under Thyr.
- Mental aberration dating three years before onset of myxedema subject to attacks of great violence, with intervals of depression and moroseness.
- State of idiocy; fearful nightmares.
- Very excited; excited state followed by considerable depression.
- Irritable and ill-tempered.
- Became a grumbler.
- Angry.
- Had frights.

Head

- Vertigo.
- Feeling of lightness in the brain, scarcely amounting to giddiness.

- Much giddiness and headache for twenty-four hours.
- Awoke about 4 a.m. with sharp headache and intense aching in back and limbs, which continued for three days and compelled him to keep his bed.

  (Constant headache, pains in occiput and vertex).

  (Headache in case of acromegaly).
- Headache.
- In one case of scleroderma and one case of myxedema the hair fell off permanently.
- In case of myxedema the patient lost all the hair of his head and face and had a thick growth over his arms and thorax; under Thyr. The hair of the head and face grew again and that of the arms and chest fell off.

Eyes

(Prominence of eyeballs—exophthalmic goitre).

- Optic neuritis (in five persons, four of them women, under treatment for obesity; no other symptoms of thyroidism).
- Accommodative asthenopia.

Ears

- Moist patches behind ears heal up (case of psoriasis). Hyperplastic median otitis with sclerosis and loss of mobility of the ossicles (rapid amelioration—several cases).

Face

- Flushing; with nausea and lumbar pains; loss of consciousness, tonic muscular spasms; immediate with rise of temperature, and pains all over; suddenly became breathless and livid.

- Faintness with great flushing of upper part of body and pains in back.
- Swelling of face and legs.
- Burning sensation of lips with free desquamation.

Mouth
- Tongue became thickly coated.
- Feverish and thirsty.
- Great thirst.

  (Ulcerated patch on buccal aspect on left cheek near angle of mouth).

Throat
- Goitre, exophthalmic, cured.

Stomach
- Loss of appetite.
- Increased appetite with improved digestion.
- Eructations.
- Dyspeptic troubles.
- Nausea, with flushing and lumbar pains.
- Always felt a sensation of sickness after the injections.
- Sensation of faintness and nausea (after a few injections).
- Gastro-intestinal disturbance and diarrhea.

Abdomen
- Flatulence increased, followed later in the case by amelioration.
- Headache and pain in abdomen.

Stool
- Diarrhea, with gastro-intestinal disturbance.
- Constipation.

Urinary Organs
- Increase flow of urine.
- Albuminuria.
- Diabetes mellitus; caused and cured.

Female Sexual Organs
- Increased sexual desire.
- Menses profuse, prolonged, more frequent; early amenorrhea.

  (Painful irregular menstruation).

  (Constant left ovarian pain, and great tenderness).
- Acts as a galactagogue when milk is deficient; when a deficiency is associated with a return of the menses it will suppress the latter.

  (Puerperal insanity with fever).

  (Puerperal eclampsia).

Respiratory Organs
- Dormant phthisis; lighted up the disease in five cases.

Heart and Pulse
- Death, with all symptoms of angina pectoris.
- Frequent fainting fits.
- Sensation of faintness and nausea.
- Palpitation on stooping.

   (Rapid pulsation, with inability to lie down in bed).

   (Jumping sensation at heart).

Back
- Stabbing pains in lumbar region.
- Flushing of upper part of body and pains in back.

Upper Limbs
- Arms less stiff and painful (psoriasis).

Lower Limbs
- Tingling sensation in legs.
- Edema of legs appeared, and subsequently subsided and continued to reappear and subside for a month.
- Pain in legs.
- Incomplete paraplegia.
- Swelling of face and legs.
- Profuse flow of fluid from feet (in case of dropsy cured by Thyr.).
- Intense aching in back and limbs, lasting three days.
- Pains in arms and legs, with malaise.
- Skin in hands and feet desquamated.

   (Acromegaly, subjective symptoms).

Generalities

- Malaise > by lying in bed.
- Stooping — palpitation.
- Rest in recumbent position > extreme breathlessness with lividity, felt as if dying.
- Myxedematous patients are always chilly; the effect of the treatment is to make them less so.
- Loss of consciousness and general tonic muscular spasm for a few seconds.
- Fainting attacks (many cases).
- Tremors, quivering of limbs, complete unconsciousness.
  (Tetany).
- Epileptiform fit, after which he was unconscious for an hour; next day felt better and warmer.
- Malaise so great she refused to continue the treatment.
- Hysterical attack.
  (Hystero-epilepsy with amenorrhea).
- Aching pains all over.
- Aching pains in various parts of body.
- Lost weight enormously (many cases of myxedema).
- Anemia and debility.
  (Acromegaly, headache and subjective symptoms).
  (Fractures refuse to unite).
- A peculiar cachexia more dangerous than myxedema itself.
- Syphilis, secondary, tertiary.

Skin

- Flushing of skin.
- Psoriasis: Eruption extended and increased.
- Lupus: Tight feeling, heat, angry redness removed; suppuration increased.
- Eczema: Irritation of skin markedly allayed.
  (Teething eczema).
  (Syphilitic psoriasis).
  (Rupia).
- Scleroderma.
- Peeling of skin of lower limbs, with gradual clearing (eczema).
- Skin of hands and feet desquamated.

Sleep

- Continual tendency to sleep.
- Insomnia.
- Excited condition; could not sleep.

Fever

- Flushing; with nausea with loss of consciousness
- Profuse perspiration on least exertion.

USTILAGO

Ustilago Maydis   *Corn-smut*

Mind
- Depression of spirits in afternoon.
- Very sad, cries frequently; exceedingly prostrated from sexual abuse and loss of semen; sleep restless.
- The day seemed like a dream.
- Melancholia; depression of spirits; oppression and faintness in a warm room. Aversion to or < from warmth in general.
- Partial or complete loss of control over the functions of vision and deglutition.
- Great irritability, mental weakness and depression.

Head
- Vertigo at climaxis with too frequent and profuse menstruation.
- Nervous headache from menstrual irregularities in nervous women.
- Bursting congestive sensation to the head; and various parts of the body.
- Feeling of fullness with dull pressive headache < by walking.
- The headache and vertigo appear to be reflex from ovarian or uterine condition.
- Frontal headache, < by walking.
- Falling of the hair and nails; complete alopecia not a hair on the head.
- Headache in temples.

Eyes
- Spasms, with vanishing of vision and head seems to whirl.
- Aching in eyes and lachrymation.
- Aching and smarting in eyeballs, with profuse secretion of tears.
- Weakness of eyes.
- Dull aching pain in right eyeball.

Nose
- Bright epistaxis. > pressure.

Face
- Burning of face, scalp from congestion.

Teeth
- Sometimes looseness of teeth.
- Aching all day in decayed upper first and second molars, which have ached before.

Mouth
- Salivation; thin, bitter; profuse.
- Taste: Coppery; in morning; slimy coppery.
- Slimy; slimy with burning distress in stomach.

Appetite
- Appetite: Craving; poor.
- Thirst at night.
- Loss of appetite followed by canine hunger.

Stomach
- Eructations: Of sour fluid; of sour food.

- Cutting in stomach.
- Pain in epigastrium with drawing pain in joints of fingers.
- Hematemesis: Passive, venous, accompanied by nausea, which is > by vomiting.
- Weak, empty, all-gone sensation in the stomach.
- Constant distress in religion of stomach.
- Burning distress in sternum and stomach, accompanied by fine neuralgic pains in same region, lasting about three minutes at a time; come on every ten or fifteen minutes for several hours; sharp cutting pain in stomach.

Abdomen
- Periodical cutting in umbilical and hypogastric regions at 6 p.m., < at 8 p.m. by a constipated stool, afterwards grumbling pain in whole abdomen.
- Pain in right lobe of liver; in umbilicus; in umbilicus before natural stool; in left groin when walking.
- Grumbling pains in abdomen all afternoon, followed by dry, hard stool, fine cutting colicky pains every few minutes all day, > by hard constipated stool, followed by dull distress in bowels.

Stool
- Light-colored diarrhea.
- Constipated: Black, dry, lumpy stools.

Urinary Organs
- Tenesmus of bladder and incontinence of urine.

Male Sexual Organs

- Spermatorrhea after onanism; emissions every night, talking about woman causes an emission; very sad; cries frequently; say he cannot break off habit, has no control of himself when passion is aroused; knows it is fast killing him; cannot work, is so prostrated.
- Genitals relaxed.
- Erections: When reading at 4 o'clock; frequently during day and night.
- Scrotum relaxed and cold sweat on it.
- Pain in testes, < right.
- Desire depressed.
- Chronic orchitis, irritable testicle.
- Erotic fancies.
- Seminal emissions and irresistible tendency to masturbation. Irresistible tendency to onanism; frequent emissions; is prostrated, dull, with lumbar backache. Despondent; irritable.
- Irritable weakness and relaxation of the male sexual organs with erotic fancies and seminal emissions.

Female Sexual Organs

- Yellow and offensive leucorrhea.
- Tenderness of left ovary, with pain and swelling.
- Burning distress in ovaries.
- Intermittent neuralgia of left ovary; enlarged, very tender to touch.
- Uterus: Hypertrophied; prolapsus; cervix sensitive, spongy.

USTILAGO

- Menses: Too scanty with ovarian irritation; too profuse and too early; blood clotted; as if everything would come through.
- Between periods constant suffering under left breast at margin of ribs.
- Oozing of dark blood, highly coagulated, forming occasionally long, black, stringy clots.
- Extreme pain during period; flow very profuse and did not cease entirely until next period; most of time confined to bed.
- Suppression of menses.
- Vicarious menstruation from lungs and bowels.
- Constant aching distress at mouth of womb.
- Menorrhagia at climaxis; active and constant flowing with frequent clots.
- Bland leucorrhea.
- Abortion.
- Deficient labor pains; of soft, pliable dilatable.
- Lochia too profuse, partly fluid, partly clotted; prolonged bearing down pains; uterus feels drawn into a knot.
- Hypertrophy and subinvolution of uterus with great atony.
- Metrorrhagia, with vertigo during climacteric.
- Menorrhagia, with displaced uterus.
- Flabby, relaxed condition of pelvic organs, a tonic condition of uterus; a state of weakness, relaxation and atony.

- Flushes of heat, and disturbances of circulation similar to those occurring at the climaxis, or from premature suppression of the menses; ovaries inflamed, irritable, sensitive and swollen; burning distress in both ovaries.
- Metrorrhagia after miscarriage, confinement or at the climaxis.
- Discharge of blood on the slightest provocation; after digital or mechanical examination; cervix swollen; bleeding easily when touched.
- Uterus remains large after miscarriage or confinement; subinvolution delayed.
- Hemorrhage bright-red but more frequently dark, clotted and stringy; post-partum oozing from flabby atonic uterus.
- Uterus hypertrophied, heavy, feels soft, spongy or boggy.
- Complaints of the lying-in woman; profuse debilitating lochia.
- Milk deficient or superabundant; nursing increases the lochial discharge.
- Acute pain < in left ovary, with swelling; pains intermittent; shoot rapidly down legs.
- Ovaritis, constant pains in ovary, sharp pains passing down legs rapidly; ovary much swollen and tender, with scanty menstruation.
- Ovaritis; took cold after menstruation; constant dull pain in right groin and back, three or four times an

hour; sharp neuralgic pain in ovary; walking painful; bowels torpid, very languid.

- Ovarian irritation, constant pain in left ovary passing down hip, has to limp when walking; pains sharp and at times pass down leg with great rapidity; every few days has quite a swelling in left groin; cannot bear pressure over ovary.

- Displaced uterus with menorrhagia; cervix tumefied; bleeds when touched.

- Uterus hypertrophied, sensitive; blood bright, fresh, without coagula.

- Subserous or interstitial fibroid of uterus (two cases), fibroid much diminished.

- Cervix tumefied, bleeds when touched.

- For days oozing of dark blood with small coagula; uterus enlarged, cervix tumefied or dilated.

- Chronic uterine hemorrhge, and passive congestion.

- Blood dark, but so thin as to scarcely color fingers.

- Profuse menstruation, flow lasting from ten days to two weeks, at first very abundant, gradually wearing off; always < from motion; discharge dark and quite painless.

- Menses every three weeks, with dark coagulum; profuse, with gushes of bright-red blood when rising from a seat or after having been startled or frightened; two days before menses, a heavy backache with sharp pain across abdomen from hip to hip, followed by expulsive pains; pains diminish

USTILAGO

after flow commence and stops with it; between menstrual periods heavy dragging backache on exertion; pain shooting up back from hips to shoulder; abdomen tender to touch; excessive bearing down; pressure in head; sensation of contraction in vertex, and feeling as if head were lifting off; vertigo; excoriating albuminous leucorrhea, < before menses; ravenous appetite; excessive tired feeling; pulse 80 and weak; mental depression.

- Subject to profuse menstruation; childless; large, fleshy, flabby, bloated-looking, with a very sallow complexion, inclined to be (and formerly had been) dropsical from excessive loss of blood; profuse menstruation, which seems to her to be principally water and clots; says there is no outward flow when she lies still, but clots and water pass out of uterus when she gets up; feels so fully in uterus that she must rise to get rid of clots; flowed fearfully during night; very low, scarcely able to speak aloud.

- Severe menorrhagia for past twelve years at every menstrual period, lasting a week or ten days, sometimes longer; pale, thin, weak, very nervous.

- Profuse discharge of dark, clotted blood of fetid odor, with pain and tenderness in one or both ovaries.

- Dysmenorrhea of a congestive character, with much ovarian irritation; severe pain in ovaries, uterus and back every few minutes; scanty, pale flow accompanied by false membranes; poor appetite, thickly-coated tongue.

- Subject to headaches ever since menstruation appeared at age of fifteen; headache mostly on top of head; appetite poor; pain in left chest with some cough; total suppression of menses for last eight months; severe pain in back, is unable to ride in carriage; pain in uterine region, especially over ovarian region, < left side; vomiting of mucus and blood daily; no sleep; some leucorrhea; hysterical; no uterine displacement, but great congestion in pelvic region.

- Suppression of menses without apparent cause; troublesome cough; considerable expectoration; sometimes also dry cough; stitching pains in chest, especially left side; night sweats; loss of appetite; pain in ovaries, especially left; general debility, headache; leucorrhea; chlorotic; anemic, as if in first stage of consumption.

- Menses suppressed for last fourteen months; very irritable and depressed; uneasiness in region of stomach; pain in ovarian region; especially left; skin hot and dry; constipation, stool dry and hard; no appetite; stitching pains in chest, < worse in left side; constant hacking cough; considerable expectoration; night sweats; general prostration; great uneasiness in lower extremities.

- Climaxis: Vertigo; frequent flushing; metrorrhagia.

Pregnancy, Parturition, Lactation

- Abortion; bearing-down pains, as if everything would come from her; in flabby constitutions; from general atony of uterus; with or without hemorrhage.

- Has aborted a number of times at third month; is now about three months pregnant; for last ten days has had more or less hemorrhage every day, some days quite bad; not so much at night; blood passes a number of times through day, in dark-colored clots.
- Post-partum hemorrhages from a flabby, atonic condition of uterus.
- Constant flooding; every few minutes, expulsion of a large clot of bright red blood, with bearing-down pains.
- Persistent hemorrhage of brownish blood, with want of uterine contraction.
- One and a half hours after delivery commenced to flow violently.
- Passive hemorrhage after miscarriage, blood in lumps, flooding for days and weeks.
- Severe flooding two weeks after labor; large bright-red clots; no pain; very weak.
- Very profuse lochial discharge, very dark in color, almost black.
- Agalactia; chronic inflammation, and induration of mamma.
- Galactorrhea.
- Promotes expulsion of foreign bodies from the uterus.
- Puerperal peritonitis; with constant flooding; high fever; secretion putrid; abdomen excessively tender and tympanitic.

- Puerperal peritonitis; aborted about two days since, at about three months; constant fever; pulse 120; cannot bear least pressure on any portion of bowels; about six times today has had sharp, cutting pains in left ovary; has flowed constantly for two days; blood dark, not copious, not attended with bearing-down pains; cannot move in bed; is compelled to lie upon her back; constant, dull, frontal headache; loss of appetite, tongue furred.
- Fibroids and induration of os.
- Discharge of blood from uterus, bright red, partly fluid, partly clotted; passive congestion of uterus, so that there is a slight oozing of blood after each examination; tissues of uterus feel soft and spongy, os patulous.

Chest
- Drawing pain in left inframmary region, waking me at 3 a.m., > turning on back from right side.

Heart
- Burning pain in cardiac region.

Respiratory Organs
- Feeling as if there were a lump behind larynx, which produces constant inclination to swallow.

Back
- Pain in back extending to extreme end of spine.
- Severe rheumatic pain in lumbar region, < by walking; aching distress in small of back.
- Pain in back of neck.

- Pain in region of right kidney, < sitting still; next day in region of left kidney, > moving about, with heat, fullness, soreness on deep pressure (but it relieved the pain), with uneasiness in left thigh, frequent desire to urinate, stream very small, the following day it requires considerable effort of will to empty the bladder, which is done slowly, pain and soreness in left loin continues; heavy in lumbar region, in bed with uneasiness about bladder (had no desire to urinate on going to bed), woke early in morning with distended feeling in bladder, micturition slow and difficult, urine scarcely colored, pain in back < next night, < lying on face, > lying on right side.
- Bearing-down in sacral region as in dysmenorrhea, changing to left ovarian region and gradually extending through hip.

Upper Limbs
- Pain in both shoulders, especially in raising arms.
- Pain in shoulder joint; rheumatic, in muscles of right shoulder, all night.
- Intermittent, numb, tingling sensation in right arm and hand every day.
- Pain in right elbow, < by motion.
- Rheumatic drawing pain in finger joints, < second joint of right index, all afternoon.
- Hypertrophy or loss of nails.
- Rheumatic pains in arms, hands and fingers.

Lower Limbs
- Pain in left knee when walking, increasing to cramp, obliging him to lean upon the arm of a friend; the pain, with occasional cramps, lasted all the evening, < raising foot so as to press upon toes.
- Cramp-like stiffness in left leg, < raising foot so as to press upon toes.
- Rheumatic pains in legs.
- Flying rheumatic pains in metatarsal bones of right foot.
- Great pains in bones all over body, and especially in calves which are somewhat cramped.

Skin
- Tendency to small boils.
- Boils on nape.
- Skin dry and hot; congested.
- Painful, destructive disease of nails.
- Paraesthesia of the skin; pricking, burning, itching, a marked erythema of skin of the uncovered parts of the body, followed by, a parchment-like, dark brown skin with rhagades < by warmth.
- Copper-colored spots on skin; secondary syphilis; macula.
- Negro, urticaria of six years' standing, troubled more or less all the time; every night itching, scratching parts produce large pale welts on body, arms and legs.

Sleep
- Difficult falling asleep and then unpleasant dreams.
- Sexual dreams; without emission; and disgusting, waking him, arose and urinated with difficulty and tenesmus.

Fever
- Chills running up and down back.
- Heat at night, during sleep.
- Internal heat; with vertigo; < eyes, which are inflamed and sensitive to light, eyeball sore to touch; intermittent; pulse normal.

Generalities
- Neuralgic pains in forehead, hands and feet.
- Rheumatic pains all up and down left side, with cutting in left knee and calf if I pressed any weight upon toes or flexed knee with any weight upon it.

Relations
- *Compare:* Meli., Med., Mez., Psor., Vinc-m., in crusta lactea and other scalp affections of childhood; Bry., Ham., Mill., Phos., in vicarious menstruation; Agar., Murx., Sep., in bearing-down and uterine collapse; Helon., Lyss., Sec., delayed subinvolution; Malan., Sec., affections of the hair and nails; Caul., Cimic., Thuj., Sulph., Vib-o., in left ovarian pain; Bov., Elaps, Graph., Ham., in intermittent flow; Sang., Urt-u., pain and rheumatic affections of right shoulder; Sang., left inframammary pain extending to scapulae; Lac-c., Kali-bi., Puls., erratic rheumatic pains; Sulph., faint all gone sensation at 11 a.m.; Cob.,

backache and seminal emissions; Bov., flow midway between the periods; Canth., Pyrog., Sec., in expelling from the uterus.

VACCININUM

A Nosode from Vaccine Matter

Mind
- Crying.
- Ill-humor, with restless sleep.
- Nervous depression, impatient, irritable; disposition to be troubled by things.
- Morbid fear of taking small pox.
- Confusion, she does not remember things at the time she wants them.

Head
- Frontal headache.
- Forehead felt as if it would split in two in median line from root of nose to top of head.
- Stitches in right temple.
- Severe headache all over head.
- Prickling in left temple, as if going to sleep.

Eyes
- Tinea tarsi and conjunctivitis in a woman, age, 28, remaining as result of variola in infancy, conjunctiva painfully sensitive.

VACCININUM

- Weak eyes; falling out in forehead as if it were split.
- Keratitis after vaccination.
- Pain in forehead and eyes as if split.
- Gauzy sensation before eyes in morning, cannot see well.

Nose
- Full feeling of head, with running of nose.
- Bleeding at nose preceded by feeling of contraction above and between eyebrows, soon after eating meat; menses rather profuse and too frequent; cured by revaccination.

Neck
- Swelling of the neck under right ear (parotid gland) with sensation like being cut.

Face
- Redness and distension of face, chill running down back, till afternoon.

Mouth
- Dry mouth and tongue.

Appetite
- Appetite gone, disgust to taste, smell, and appearance of food.
- Coffee tastes sour.
- Good appetite.

Stomach
- Aching in pit of stomach, with short breath.

Abdomen
- A stitch in hepatic region, at margin in last lower rib, axillary line.
- Stitch in splenic region.
- Blown up with flatulence.

Urinary Organs
- Nephritis with albuminuria, hematuria, and dropsy, developed eleven days after vaccination; child recovered.

Respiratory Organs
- Whooping cough.

Chest
- Stitches in right side under short ribs in front from right to left then a corresponding place left side, but from left to right, lasting five minutes, felt in liver and spleen.

Heart
- Aching at heart.

Bach
- Backache.
- Aching pain in back, < in lumbar region extending around waist.
- Twisting pain in lower back.
- Weakness in small of back coming on suddenly, > by lying down.

Upper Limbs
- Rheumatic pains in wrists and hands.

Lower Limbs

- Soreness of lower extremities, as if heated or over-exerted.
- Twisting pains in both knees.

Skin

- A general eruption similar to cow pox.
- Small pimples develop at point of vaccination with fourth dilution.
- Red pimples or blotches in various parts, most evident when warm.
- Eruption of pustules with a dark red base and roundish or oblong elevation, filled with pus of a greenish-yellow color, at left side of trunk, between shoulder, on left shoulder, behind right ear, resembling varioloid, some as large as a pea, some less without depression in the centre, coming with a round, hard feel in the skin (like a shot), very itchy.
- Vaccininum 200th quickly > severer symptoms of variola occurring in a child, age, six months; two days before appearance of eruption had been revaccinated (after an interval of eight days) on a nevus near right nipple; deglutition difficult through implication of tongue and fauces; pustules, many of large size, scattered over scalp, face, body and limbs.
- Eruption of small, red vesicles on left upper arm and chest dying off after a few days.
- Pustule filled with matter, with a depression in centre and red halo on left shoulder.
- Pustules suddenly much depressed.

- Eruption all over body of small pustules, some with a central depression, some brown.

Generalities
- Restlessness.
- General malaise.
- Languor, lassitude.
- Tired all over, with stretching, gaping feeling; unnatural fatigue.
- Child wants to be carried.
- Many persons faint when being vaccinated.
- Weakness.

PROVINGS OF THE X-RAY

Mind and Disposition
- Mental irritability.
- Clearing up of mental function after sharp stabbing pain in left temple staggering him, the heart feeling the impulse immediately.
- Mental processes not clear, writes wrong words in letters.
- Mental condition upset during profuse menstruation, would like to kill somebody.

Head
- Sleepy with headache.

- Headache gradually extending to frontal region, worse in centre of forehead.
- Sense of pressure in centre of forehead.
- Dull headache in morning, worse when stooping and after rising.
- Headache and soreness, worse towards afternoon.
- Head feels empty as though scraped, worse at night in bed.
- Pain in right side of head above temple.
- Sharp stabbing in left temple, followed by clearing up of mental function, the heart immediately feeling the impulse.
- Sense of pressive fullness starting from posterior prominence of vertex in a central straight line to bridge of nose, followed by fullness in entire vertex extending to bridge of nose.
- Aggravation of fullness over vertex, worse along the centre to nose and when stooping over.
- Aching on top of head across a long coronal suture on blowing nose and after it.
- Constant ache in vertex, worse on awaking; also on coughing, sneezing, or head low.
- Heavy pressure on vertex as from a hand (old symptom, absent a year).
- Sticking pains in different parts of head and face.
- Cannot bear slightest touch though hard pressure relieves for an instant; > by walking the floor.

- Pain > by lying on left side of face and body.
- Pain in back of head > at times by massage slightly, also by heat.
- Neuralgic pains.

Neck
- Stiffness on left side of neck, turning in bed.
- Stiffness on right side of neck, with intense pain at night; occurs in paroxysms during the day > somewhat by hot applications.
- Sudden "cricks" attack first on side of neck, then the other, < on getting cold; turning the head nearly produces convulsions. Pains more severe behind the ears—the mastoid process.
- Pain relieved on keeping perfectly quiet; sometimes by gentle stinging contraction pain.

Eyes
- Eyeballs sore.
- Sensation in right eye as if bulging.

Ears
- Fullness in ears, worse in right ear, worse by inserting finger.
- Intermittent noise as of deep steam-whistle in left ear, and ringing in head.
- Ears more clear from ringing and dullness of hearing than for many years, an improvement lasting up to this day. Healing action.

Nose
- Bloody mucus from the nose.
- Sulphur vapor sensation in throat and nose.
- Congested sensation in head and nose as before coryza.

Face
- Slight electric current sensation in left side of tongue and face passing over and disappearing in right side of face.

Mouth
- Tongue dry, rough, sore and scraped.
- Scrapping pain in lateral incisor, aggravated by noises and jarring of cars.

Throat
- Sulphur vapor sensation in nose and throat.
- Throat painful on swallowing.

Appetite
- Aversion to meat.
- Appetite diminished.
- Desire for sweets.
- Most distress after midday and evening meal.
- No hunger, goes till he feels faint.
- Can eat plenty but does not enjoy it.
- More thirst than usual.
- Thirst for cold drinks though nothing tastes good.
- Bad taste in forenoon.
- Bitter taste.

Nausea, Vomiting
- Nausea and vomiting with profuse sweat after immense stool at 4 a.m., seven days after taking.

Abdomen
- Abdomen distended with full feeling (Pulsatilla, which a year ago helped for months a train of symptoms, had only very slight effect).
- Flatulence with ineffectual desire for stool.
- Colicky pains in right lower abdomen, sometimes extending behind the hip, and retained urine.

Stool
- Stools green, though normal in consistency.
- On straining at stool a sore sensation in nates.
- Ineffectual urging of stool, with flatulence.

Urine
- Retained urine, vesical tenesmus after enormous evacuation, vomiting for twelve hours to 4 p.m.
- Frequent urination, worse after getting into bed.
- Pressure as from congestion about kidneys.

Male Sexual Organs
- Sexual desire lost in man.
- Testes relaxed, impotent feeling.
- Unnatural or disgusting, lewd dreams on several nights, or several times in one night.

Female Sexual Organs
- Menses dark green one day.

- Pain darting upward in region of left ovary when sitting, walking or standing.
- Flushes of heat; better afternoons and evenings.

Chest
- Wandering; sticking pains in chest, worse on right side.
- Stitching pain in right upper chest going through to upper part of scapula.

Heart
- Palpitation during evening causing cough.
- Sharp pain at apex of heart, better by lying on left side.
- Palpitation with a cough with tearing sensation in bronchi and hoarseness.
- Heart's sound keeps him awake while lying on left side.
- Dull and constant soreness around heart, and worse in legs and arms.

Back
- Pain in dorsal region.
- Lame and stiff in back.
- Aching whole length of spine.
- A paralytic sensation extending from spine down left leg.
- Rheumatic-like fever in trunk, steady dull pain going steadily from trunk to legs, and finally to heels, worse in left knee, worse stepping on heel, on

underside of heel (old symptom of inflammatory rheumatism twenty-five years ago).

Upper Extremities
- Rheumatic pain in left wrist and forearm.
- Rheumatic twinge in last two phalangeal articulations of index and middle fingers for a short time in forenoon.
- Grating heard in shoulder joints, as well as nearly all other joints of the body.
- Rheumatic pain in right wrist and arm.
- Can't hold things in left hand, powerless or clumsy.
- Palms of hands, which where rough and scaly and bleeding at times, became smooth and natural during the proving. Healing action. (Afterward they went back to former state when general health improved.)

Lower Extremities
- Lower part of both legs asleep, tingling as if from electric battery more in right, immediately.
- Sciatic pain in right hip.
- Rheumatic pains in limbs.
- Dull aching posterior aspect of thigh and calf in morning, from above downward.
- Pain in right sciatic nerve on walking.
- Rheumatic pains in front of right thigh.
- Drawing aching discomfort in right thigh through hip and knees down through toes, immediately.

- Feeling as if somebody were drawing icy hands over thigh downward, aggravatingly slow. (This occurred first twelve years ago after a nervous shock and did not return for five years.)
- Rheumatic-like fever in trunk, steady dull pain going steadily down to legs and finally to heels, worse in left knee, worse stepping on heel, on underside of heel (old symptoms of inflammatory rheumatism twenty-five years ago).

Fever
- Chills as soon as beginning to sleep, running up back, preventing sleep.
- Chill going down back, followed by paralytic feeling in right cheek.
- Wave-like sensation as if it would break out in perspiration.
- Profuse perspiration on getting into bed, keeping him awake.

Sleep
- Keep awake by heart's sound while lying on left side.
- As soon as she begins to sleep, chills running up back preventing sleep.
- Sleeplessness constant and troublesome (relieved permanently by a bottle of Pabst Malt Extract).
- Drowsy all night while sitting up.
- Drowsiness leaves the instant when laying down, so cannot sleep.

- Symptoms worse when getting into bed, worse after sunset.
- Profuse perspiration on getting on getting into bed, keeping him awake.
- Sleepy during day.
- Walking frequently at night from no apparent cause.
- All symptoms worse in bed.
- Dreams of strife, busy dreams.
- Very vivid lewd dreams, repeated night after night.

General Symptoms
- General tired and sick feeling.
- Persistent exhaustion and languor, not attributable to spring.
- Lame and sore all over.
- Trembling all over.

Skin
- Reappearance of an old, slight, pimply eruption on left side of forehead.
- Return of a slight eruption on outside of lower legs, burning when scratched, worse after scratching.

Relation
Compare: The Calcareas, Caust., Hep., Med., Nat-m., Psor., Puls., Sil., Sulph., Thuj., Tub., for its power to reproduce old or suppressed symptoms and conditions; Cimic., Lac-c., Lil-t., Plat., Sep., Pyrog., for nervous reflexes and neuralgic conditions from ovarian or uterine irritation: Agar., Cur., Tarent.,

Zinc., for irritation of the cord, spinal reflexes, neurasthenia; electric storms, thunderstorms, Agar., Med., Nat-c., Phos., Psor., Rhod., Sep., Sil., Syph., Thuj.

Antidotes

Nux-v., Sulph. and the dynamic potencies of the remedy.

Aggravation

In bed; towards evening and at night (both mental and physical); in the open air; in the afternoon.

THE BOWEL NOSODES

By John Paterson M.B., Ch.B., D.P.H. (Camb.) F.F. Hom.

INTRODUCTION

The name of one of your illustrious countrymen, Louis Pasteur, will forever be remembered as the founder of the science of bacteriology. It was he who first isolated and identified a specific germ and related it to a definite clinical entity (disease). Following upon his discoveries, medical science concentrated on the laboratory technique for the isolation and identification of a specific germ for each known disease, and the Koch postulates were accepted as the standard of declaring any germ capable of pathogenesis – of having power to cause disease. The motto of the medical profession is still *Tolle Causum*, find the cause, and today there are many who consider that germs are the only cause of disease and are working to discover the specific germ of virus for well known clinical entities.

It must now be accepted as a scientific fact that specific germs, in many cases of disease, can be isolated and identified, but is it a true conclusion that the specific germ is always the cause of the disease? The subject is too great to be dealt with in all its aspects in this short session, but a little time must be given to consider the general question, namely the role of the Bacterium in nature because one's opinion on this must determine the value one places on the use of bacterial products— vaccines or nosodes—in the treatment of disease. As the subject of this paper deals with the intestinal flora, I propose to limit my remarks to consideration of the role played by the *B. Coli* and coliform organisms found in the intestinal tract.

The role of the intestinal bacteria B. Coli can be isolated from the intestine of all warm blooded animals and have been found on grasses outside the body, where there seemed to be no possibility of fecal contamination. Most workers consider the *B. Coli* to be a *harmless* saprophyte and to be non-pathogenic in the healthy bowel. Its function is to break up into the more simple substances the complex molecules of the organic combinations which form the bodies of plants and animals, or of the complex substances which result from the digestive processes in the intestinal canal and are excreted. It is important to note this function in the further study of the intestinal flora and its relationship to disease.

In nature, where there is balance, there is no *disease* and the germ, in this case, the *B. Coli* in the intestinal tract, performs a useful function. Where the intestinal

---

[*] Read to the Rodanienne Homoeopathic Society at the Meeting of the International Homoeopathic League Council, August, 1949.

mucosa is healthy, the *B. Coli* is non-pathogenic. Any change in the host which affects the intestinal mucosa will upset the balance and will be followed by a change in the habit and the biochemistry of the *B. Coli*, which may then be said to become pathogenic, but it should be noted that the primary change, the *dis-ease* originated in the host, which compelled the bacillus to modify its habit in order to survive, I would ask you to keep this sequence of events in mind as a great deal of what I have to say about the intestinal nosodes is based upon this conception which I have a confirmed by clinical and laboratory observations over the last twenty years.

In 1936 I presented a paper to the British Homoeopathic Society, which was published in their Journal of April, 1936, under the title of "The potentised Drug and its Action on the Bowel Flora" and it dealt with the clinical and bacteriological observations on 12,000 cases. A brief summary of the findings is as follows:

(a) Non-lactose fermenting bacilli were isolated in 25 percent of the stool specimens examined.

(b) The appearance of non-lactose fermenting bacilli often *followed* and seemed to bear relationship to the previously administered homoeopathic remedy—the choice of the remedy being made according to the law of similars" and prepared by "potentization".

In the laboratory one observed an unexpected phenomenon, that from a patient who had previously yielded only *B. Coli*, there suddenly appeared a large percentage of non-lactose fermenting bacilli of a type which one associated with the pathogenic group of typhoid and paratyphoid.

If one accepts the view, generally held, that the *B. Coli* of the intestinal tract is a harmless saprophyte and is non-pathogenic it must be concluded that, so far as the intestinal tract was concerned there was no evidence of disease in these patients during the first series of examinations. Now the patient's stool yielded a large percentage of presumably pathogenic organisms, and according to the accepted Pasteur and Koch theory, the patient was suffering from disease. Clinical investigations, however, revealed that the patient did not feel ill, but had experienced a sense of well being which he had attributed to the last medicine he had received. Since the non-lactose fermenting bacilli had appeared after a definite latent period of 10 to 14 days, following the administration of the remedy, it would seem that the *homoeopathic potentized remedy* had changed the bowel flora, and had caused the *dis-ease*. The pathogenic germ in this case was the result of vital action set up in the patient by the potentized remedy, the germ was *not* the *cause* of the disease.

Is the "specific germ" the actual cause of *dis-ease*, or is it the result of the action of the vital force (dynamis) which characterizes all living cells, in their resistance to disease? That is a question which I must ask you to consider and answer for yourselves in the light of the observations I have placed before you today. Meantime, it will be sufficient for the purpose of continuing the subject of this paper, if we agree that each germ is associated with its own peculiar symptom picture (disease) and that certain conclusions may be made from these clinical and laboratory observations and translated into the practice of medicine.

(a) The specific organism is related to the disease.

(b) The specific organism is *related to the homoeopathic remedy.*

(c) The homoeopathic remedy is related to the disease.

From my observations I have been able to compile a list of bowel organisms with their related homoeopathic remedies and to associate a clinical picture, i.e. to offer a "proving" for each type of bowel organism. In this case the word "proving" is not used in the strict Hahnemann sense—experiment on the healthy human—but on clinical observation of the sick person.

It is not possible to give a detailed account of each type in one session, so I propose to give you a brief summary for each, indicating a keynote, the main action. From this, and your knowledge of the associated homoeopathic remedies, you should be able to formulate a more complete picture of the symptom complex of these bowel organisms, and later I shall indicate how this knowledge can be put into practice.

MORGAN (Bach)

B. Morgan is the type of non-lactose organism most frequently found in the stool and it has the greatest number of associated remedies compared to other types on the list.

The keynote for the *Morgan* group is contained in the word *"congestion"* and if this is used in the study of the various parts of the body affected it will afford a good symptom picture of the pathogenesis of the *B. Morgan*.

Head

Congestive headaches, with flushed face; worse from hot atmosphere; thundery weather excitement; travelling in bus or train. Vertigo from high blood pressure.

Mentals

Introspective, anxious and apprehensive about state of health; irritability; avoids company but often shows mental anxiety if left alone. Mental depression, often with suicidal tendency.

Digestive System

Congetion of gastric mucosa and liver; heart-burn, pyrosis, dirty tongue, bitter taste in mouth in the morning with accumulation of mucus causing gagging as soon as rises from bed. Congestion of liver; "bilious attacks "with severe headache which is finally relieved by vomiting large quantities of bile stained mucus. (A history of "bilious attacks", especially occurring at the menopause in women should lead one to consider the use of the nosode, *Morgan* (Bach).) Cholecystitis, gallstone; constipation, hemorrhoids, pruritus ani.

Respiratory System

Congestion of nasal and bronchial membrane, especially in children, broncho and lobar pneumonia. (A history of repeated attacks of "congestion of the lungs or broncho-pneumonia," in children, is indicative for the use of the nosode *Morgan* (Bach) or one of the sub-types *Morgan Pure* (Paterson) or *Morgan Gaertner* (Paterson).

It is worth noticing, in view of the frequent use of the Sulpha drugs in the treatment of pneumonia, that *Sulphur* is outstanding among the remedies associated with *Bacillus Morgan* of the intestinal tract.

Female Reproductive System

The congestive headache associated with the menstrual onset has already been mentioned, and this is often accompanied by ovarian pain (congestive dysmenorrhea) or by the congestive flushing of the menopause period.

Circulation

Congestion and sluggish action is seen by the tendency to hemorrhoids and varicose veins and the condition known as "erythro-cyanosis puellorum", a blueness of the lower extremities, often in female adolescents and marked by chilblains of feet and toes.

Fibrous Tissues

Chronic congestion around the joints causes arthritic conditions, usually affecting the phalangeal or knee joint regions.

Skin

It is here that the outstanding action of the *Bacillus Morgan* group of organisms is to be found. *Morgan* (Bach) is the nosode indicated where there is congestion of the skin with itching eruption, worse from heat. The type of eruption which characterizes this can be ascertained from a study of the "provings" of well known skin remedies found among the list of remedies associated with the *Bacillus Morgan,* e.g. *Sulphur, Graphites, Petroleum* and *Psorinum.* There are few eczemas of the infant at teething stage or later life, which do not require a dose of the nosode *Morgan* (Bach). It was found possible to isolate two sub-types of *Bacillus Morgan* and to observe the clinical indications for the use of the respective nosodes.

1. *Morgan Pure* (Paterson) is indicated where there is a marked symptom of skin eruption or disturbance of the liver; bilious headache, or actual presence of gallstones.

2. *Morgan Gaertner* (Paterson) is also indicated in skin and liver conditions, but it is likely to be more useful where there is evidence of acute inflammatory attack, such as the found in cholecystitis.

The sub-type *Morgan Gaertner* (Paterson) has often been found in the stool of patients suffering from renal colic and where X-ray has demonstrated the presence of renal calculus. The nosode *Morgan Gaertner* (Paterson) should therefore be considered as a possible remedy in cases of renal colic. It is also likely to be of value in treatment in any case which has a 4-8 p.m. modality which is also a characteristic of the group prototype remedy—*Lycopodium*. For its prototype, *Morgan Pure* (Paterson) has Sulphur and within the main group represented by *Morgan* (Bach) you will find the well known trio of remedies mentioned by Kent as working in a cycle of *Sulphur, Calcarea* and *Lycopodium*.

PROTEUS (Bach)

It is difficult of offer you a single word with which to explain the pathogenesis of the *Bacillus Proteus,* but it will be useful at the outset to suggest to you that the nosode *Proteus* (Bach) will seldom have any therapeutic action unless there are outstanding symptoms in the case relative to the central or peripheral nervous systems and symptoms which appear with a degree of suddenness.

Mentals

Mental symptoms are prominent in the clinical proving and "brain storm" might be taken as the keynote to indicate the sudden and violent upset of the nervous system.

Outburst of violent temper, especially if opposed in any way; will throw any missile which is at hand;

kick or strike; the child objecting to parental control will lie on the; floor and kick and scream.

Emotional hysteria, suggestive of the remedy *Ignatia* is also found in the proving of the *Bacillus Proteus* preparation and convulsive and epileptiform seizures and meningismus in children during febrile attacks often responds to the action of the nosode *Proteus* (Bach) circulation. Further indication for the use of this nosode is disturbance of the peripheral nervous system, evidenced by *spasm* of the peripheral circulation, e.g. "dead fingers"; intermittent claudication in the circulation of the lower limbs; anginal attacks due to spasm of the coronary capillaries. There are two well known diseases associated with capillary spasm where the nosode *Proteus* (Bach) has been found useful in treatment—Raynaud's disease, where there is spasm of the capillary circulation of the extremities, and Meniere's disease where spasm of the brain circulation results in vertigo attacks.

Digestive System

It is important to note that many of the symptoms manifested in the digestive system are secondary to the action of the central nervous system. It is now being realized that prolonged nerve strain is a factor in the production of duoedenal ulcer, and in the *Proteus* proving, this is also to be found. The type of case is that where there are no prodromal symptoms in the digestive system and the first sign is that of a hematemesis or melena. These ulcers have a tendency to perforate, probably due to the innervation and interference with capillary circulation in that area.

As part of the scientific discussion at this meeting, a study is to be made of the remedy *Natrium muriaticum* and you will note that this is given in my list as the outstanding member to the list of remedies I associate with the *Proteus* nosode, and I may have the opportunity of further discussing with you the significance of the disturbed chloride metabolism associated with the intestinal organism.

Neuro-muscular System

As one might expect from the forgoing indications, cramp of muscles is a characteristic symptom and *Cuprum metallicum* is also found among the list of remedies.

Skin

Angio-neurotic edema, which one associates with the remedy *Apis mellifica* is found in the proving of the *Bacillus Proteus* preparation and also a tendency for the production of herpetic eruption at the muco-cutaneous margins.

There is marked sensitivity to exposure to ultra-violet light.

Before leaving this "proving" of *Proteus* (Bach), it may be of interest to you to know that in Great Britain since the war years, there has been a marked increase in the frequency with which one has been able to isolate *Bacillus Proteus*, and this I associate with long continued "nerve strain"—a factor of considerable importance of the pathogenesis of the type of bowel organism.

BACILLUS NO. "7" (Paterson)

This is so named because it was the 7th non-lactose fermenting type of bacillus to be observed in the laboratory, and as it did not conform to any to the previously known groups, it was given the numeral "7".

As a keynote for the use of this nosode I suggest *"mental and physical fatigue"*. The "proving" of *Bacillus No. "7"* is not unlike that of *Proteus* (Bach) as it has similar relationship; *Proteus* (Bach) is related to *Chlorine* whereas *Bacillus No. "7"* seems to have a closer relationship to the two halogens, *Bromine* and *Iodine*, often in combination with *Potassium*.

Mentals

The outstanding symptom is mental fatigue, a feeling of unfitness for any mental effort, which produces a sense of extreme physical exhaustion.

Digestive System

All the symptoms can be related to general lack of nerve and muscle tone; a sense of fullness after food; flatulence and distension of the stomach; enteroptosis.

Genito-urinary System

Feeble urinary flow; loss of sexual function; premature senility to raise.

Respiratory System

Asthma; bronchial catarrh; tough sticky mucus, difficult to raise.

(Compare the symptom picture of *Kalium carb.*, which is one of the associated remedies).

Circulation

Slow pulse rate, often with lowered blood pressure; myocardial weakness.

(*Potassium* has a specific action on cardiac muscle.)

Neuro-muscular System

Relaxed fibrous tissue, with tendency to the formation of "rheumatic nodules"; backache, cannot stand long without feeling of faintness; tendency to syncope after sudden exertion.

Skin

Nothing outstanding; sensitive to cold, to draughts and cold damp air.

GAERTNER (Bach)

The keynote for this nosode is *"malnutrition"* and as this would imply, it is the nosode applicable to the treatment of many diseases of childhood, but it is also found to be of value in the other extreme of life associated with malignancy. Marked emaciation may be taken as an indication for the use of the *Gaertner* nosode.

Mentals

Mostly observed in the child; hypersensitive to all impressions, psychical or physical; overactive brain with under-nourished body.

Digestion

It is in the digestive tract that the *Bacillus Gaertner* has its greatest action, and this often manifests itself about the age of 6 months at the time when the infant is put on to artificial feeding.

The inability to digest fat—*coeliac disease; ketosis; "intestinal infantilism"*—are all disease complexes found under the "proving" of the *Bacillus Gaertner* preparation; also chronic *gastro-enteritis; tabes mesenterica;* thread worms. The clearing of thread worms is difficult and usually requires prolonged treatment.

It your combine the clinical picture of three well known remedies with which you are familiar, *Phosphorus, Silicea, Mercurius vivus*, you will have before you a very good clinical picture of the "proving" of *Gaertner* (Bach).

DYS. CO. (Bach)

This is the nosode prepared *B. dysenteriae* and the keynote for its use is nervous system of a peculiar type and best described as *"anticipatory"*, since it is that sense of nerve tension which a student might feel immediately before facing his examiners, or a businessman before attending an important engagement.

Mentals

Nervous tension, mental uneasiness in anticipation of some event; hypersensitive to criticism; shyness and uneasiness among strangers; mental uneasiness shows itself by physical restlessness, cannot keep still, fidgets, choreic movements of facial muscles, or limbs. Headache, frontal over the eyes, or in vertex, brought on by excitement; often occurs at regular time periods of 7 or 14 days' cycle.

Digestive System

Bacillus Dysenteriae has been shown to have selective action on the pylorus causing spasm and retention of digested contents; dilatation of stomach; wakened at 12 midnight to 1 a.m. with acute pain in stomach, relieved by vomiting of a large quantity of mucous material.

In some children, diagnosed as suffering from *congenital pyloric stenosis* considerable success has followed the use of *Dys. Co.* (Bach), which would suggest that in these cases the condition had been due to pyloric spasm rather than to congenital malformation of the pylorus.

Duodenal ulcer often calls for the use of the nosode *Dys. Co.* (Bach) but there must always be present evidence of nervous tension, which always precedes the physical symptom and which the patient feels and refers to his "stomach and heart areas." This is in contrast to the type of duodenal ulcer found associated with *B. Proteus*, where the nerve tension is insidious in action, unperceived by the patient, and the physical condition the ulcer – tends to come on as a "crisis" without previous warning.

Cardio-vascular

Functional disturbance of heart action, associated with nerve tension; palpitation before important events; anticipatory discomfort in the cardiac area.

These are the outstanding symptoms found in the clinical proving of the nosode *Dys. co.* (Bach), and you will find in them something of each of the associated remedies, *Arsenicum album, Argentum nit., Kalmia.*

SYCOTIC CO. (Paterson)

This organism is not of bacillary form but is a non-lactose fermenting coccus found in the intestinal tract. The details of this organism and the manner in which it was identified, is to be found in the original work published in the British Homoeopathic Journal of April, 1933.

The keynote for the nosode *Sycotic co.* (Paterson) is "irritability" and this has special reference to mucous and synovial membrane.

Mentals

Nervous irritability; tempery (cf. *Lycopodium*); fear of dark; of being left alone; twitching of facial muscles, blinking of eyelids.

Head

Irritation of meninges, sub-acute or chronic; headache from infection of sinuses; persistent headache—particularly in a child—which may be the prodromal sign of a tubercular meningitis (cf-*Hellebore*); sweating of head at night, profuse.

Digestive System

Chronic irritation of the whole alimentary tract;

catarrhal conditions; acute or chronic gastroenteritis in the child; loose offensive stool excoriating (cf. *Medorrhinum)*; urgent call to stool as soon as rising out of bed; constipation unusual; diarrhea common; nausea or sickness after eating eggs (cf. *Ferrum met.*).

Respiratory

Acute, sub-acute, chronic bronchial catarrh; catarrh of mucous membranes of nose, throat (enlarged tonsils and adenoids in child). Irritable cough at night, 2 a.m.

(I regard *Sycotic co.* (Paterson) as a pre-tubercular remedy).

Circulation

Anemia and hydremia, usually in the adult.

(The sycotic patient is always anemic looking, never carries much color in the face.)

Neuro-muscular System

General rheumatic fibrositis, aggravated from dampness, after a period of rest (cf. *Rhus tox.*).

Feet painful when walking, as if walking on loose cobble stones, pain in the metarsal bones, fidgety feet at night in bed.

Skin

Sallow complexion, oily skin, vesicular or varicellar type of eruption of face or body. (After administration of *Sycotic co.* (Paterson) to children, a rash, varicellar in type, resembling, and often mistaken for chicken pox may appear.) Warts on muco-cutaneous surfaces.

Genito-urinary System

Sycotic co.(Paterson) has marked action of the whole of the genito-urinary tract causing irritation of mucous membranes from the kidney to the urethral tract; albuminuria; pyelitis; cystitis; urethritis; vulvo-vaginities; balanitis.

Female Reproductive System

Pain in left ovary at menstrual period; cystic ovaries; tubal infection (tubercular or gonococcal); profuse leucorrhea.

It will be evident that this coccal organism of the intestinal tract is related morphologically and clinically to the gonococcus. Hahnemann related what he called "the Sycotic Miasm" to the disease, gonorrhea, but this disease is only one form of catarrhal infection of the mucous membrane of the urinary tract. There are many other non-gonorrheal organisms associated with the symptom picture of "catarrh" and I suggest that the miasm "sycosis" may be considered synonymous with "catarrh". Gonorrhea is an infection of mucous membrane (i.e., it is a sycotic manifestation) but catarrhal manifestations (*Sycotic*) or not all due to gonorrheal infection.

These are the nosodes prepared from the non-lactose fermenting organisms of the bowel which are most generally called for in practice, but there are two other members which are found occasionally in the stool and which are not well proved and seldom used.

MUTABILE (Bach)

This bacillus is so named because it mutates almost as soon as it is sub-cultured from a non-lactose fermenter and is of interest mainly from a bacteriological point of view as the *Bacillus Mutabile* is an intermediary form between the *B. Coli* and the pure non-lactose fermenting type. Its associated remedy is *Pulsatilla* and the nosode *Mutabile* (Bach) is likely to be of value in treatment where there is alteration of symptoms, e.g. where skin eruption alternates with asthmatic symptoms.

FAECALIS (Bach)

I have never found this nosode made from the *B. Fecalis* of much value in treatment, but where I have found the organism in the stool, the clinical symptoms have led me to choose *Sepia* as the indicated remedy.

THE BIOCHEMISTRY OF THE BOWEL ORGANISMS AND THEIR ASSOCIATED REMEDIES

I would ask you now to refer to the list before you and to note the group remedies which have been found associated with each type of non-lactose fermenting organism of the bowel.

B. MORGAN (Bach)

In this go up two elements are outstanding i.e., *Sulphur* and *Carbon*. In this group also there are complex remedies from the plant world e.g. *Lycopodium* and from the venom of a snake, i.e. *Lachesis*.

B. PROTEUS (Bach)

Here the outstanding element is *Chlorine*.

BACILLUS NO. "7" (Paterson)

Bromine and *Iodine*.

B. GAERTNER (Bach)

Silicea; Phosphorus; Fluorine; Mercurius viv.

From this list it will be evident that each organism is associated with remedies which have a central element with which other elements may combine to form remedies of varying chemical complexity. The practice of homoeopathy is founded on the hypothesis that the true *simillimum* (the homoeopathic remedy) is related to the disturbed metabolism (the disease) and now it can be demonstrated that the non-lactose fermenting organism of the bowel is biochemically related to the disease and the homoeopathic remedy.

The potentized vaccine—the nosode—prepared from culture of the organism can be considered to be a complex biochemical substance having the characteristic of the disturbed metabolism, and thus to be similar to the disease and according to the law of similars, to have specific therapeutic power to restore balance, a condition of ease—i.e. health.

The individual members of each group may have some therapeutic action in a specific disease, but the action of the simpler elements may be incomplete and require the assistance of the more complex remedies, and on this hypothesis one can formulate a series of working rules for the use of the remedies and the nosodes and in actual practice demonstrate how one may complement the action of the other.

INDICATIONS FOR THE USE OF THE BOWEL NOSODES IN DISEASE

My remarks will be addressed, on this occasion, to those doctors who have no means of obtaining bacteriological reports on stool culture, but who may wish to try out the use of these nosodes in their practice.

I suggest that we divide the cases to be considered into two groups:

1. *New case.* A patient who has not received homoeopathic treatment.
2. *Old case.* A patient who has been under homoeopathic treatment but who may be responding to the treatment given.

In using the bowel nosodes it must always be remembered that they are deep-acting remedies and they cover the totality of symptoms from the highest level, the "mentals", to the lowest level of "gross pathology" and that they also cover the life history of a patient from earliest childhood to adult life or old age.

The "taking of the case history" is therefore of great importance in the choice of the nosode for a particular case, and attention must be given to the "past" as well as the "present" symptoms.

New Case

Where this is a definite symptom picture which points to a remedy, this should be given, and not a nosode. In many cases, however, the choice may lie within a number of possible remedies and it is in this difficulty that one may use the list of remedies and the associated bowel nosode. If, for example, *Sulphur, Calcarea carbonica, Graphites* were among the list of possible remedies, reference to the table would show that the nosode *Morgan-pure* (Paterson) was related to each of these and could be considered to cover the totality of the symptoms. In practice this is found to be so and proves the bowel nosodes to be deep and broad acting remedies.

As another example, the choice might lie within group of remedies *Mercurius viv., Phosphorus, Silicea,* in which case the nosode *Gaertner* (Bach) would be indicated.

In this way it is possible to choose the nosode from the list of possible remedies for a given case, but the next question to decide is that of potency and repetition of dose.

As in general homoeopathic practice the more obvious the "mentals" the higher the potency, but if there are marked pathological symptoms the general rule is to employ the lower potencies.

With outstanding "mentals" I prefer the nosode in *1M* potency or higher, if obtainable, but if there is obvious evidence of advanced pathological conditions such as advanced rheumatoid arthritis or malignancy, I would employ the *6c* potency and give this in a daily dose over a period, the duration of which would be determined by clinical observations and evidence of reaction.

Between these extremes there is an intermediate level of potency—*30c*—which I have found useful where there is a combination of acute and chronic, e.g. in acute broncho-pneumonia superimposed upon a chronic condition, with a miasmatic background, a tubercular diathesis.

The number and frequency of the doses of the chosen nosode can be determined only by clinical observation and experience.

The higher the potency chosen the less frequent the repetition and number of doses, is a good working rule for the use of the nosodes, but it has been found a useful practice to complement the action of a nosode in single high potency dose, with repeated doses of the low potency of an associated remedy. As example, a case of skin eruption may call for a single dose of *Morgan-pure* (Paterson) *1M* but the intolerable itch may also call for *Sulphur* in the *3x* to the *6c* potency in repeated doses. Also in chronic arthritis, after a dose of the appropriate nosode for the case, considerable benefit to the patient may follow the use of a low potency remedy, chosen from the lit of associated remedies, and given over a considerable period of time.

Old Case

This is where the patient may have had homoeopathic treatment over a period and received a considerable number of remedies with a varying degree of success or failure. These are difficult cases, even from the nosode point of view; when there is no evidence available from stool culture to give a clue to the group of remedies likely to be useful, or as to the phase in which the patient is at the moment. It must be remembered that the potentized remedy can alter the bowel flora and that in an "old case" the remedies already given may have caused a positive phase, i.e. changed the *B. Coli* to non-lactose bacilli, and consideration must be given to the extent of this change. If I find a percentage of non-lactose fermenting organisms in a stool greater than 50 percent, I at once determine that the administration of a bowel nosode is contraindicated, and experience has shown that a nosode given at such a time produces a negative phase with a corresponding period of vital depression in the patient.

With this uncertainty in an old case, which has had potentized remedies within one month, it is wise to use a nosode in the 6c potency in the first instance, and so avoid the chance of a violent negative reaction.

The choice of a nosode for any case can be determined by a study of the clinical history and noting the remedies which have given the greatest, although not sustained, effect. Tabulate this list of remedies and compare it with the nosode list and the associated remedies and choose the nosode which has the greatest number within its group. In many cases there may not be much apparent effect from the nosode, but it would seem that the giving of the nosode has in some manner readjusted the case, because thereafter considerable benefit follows the remedy previously given without much effect. If there seems no apparent benefit from the nosode, do not be disappointed but repeat the remedy which has given the evidence of partial reaction before, and this time you can expect more permanent action.

One last remark, and that of warning, do no repeat a bowel nosode within three months; but if it is necessary to prescribe, select a remedy within the group, and give the remedy in high or low potency as you find indicated from the symptoms present. Finally, do not expect too much from these bowel nosodes, and then be disappointed in their use. They are valuable therapeutic agents when properly used, and their great value is in the treatment of chronic disease, in cases which are generally considered to be very resistant to any form of treatment.

Note on Nomenclature

3x = 3rd decimal Hahnemannian.

6c = 6 centesimal Hahnemannian.

30c = 30 centesimal Hahnemannian.

1m = 1,000 centesimal Hahnemannian.

THE BOWEL NOSODES
AMENDED LIST (SEPTEMBER, 1949)

Morgan (Bach)
  (a) Morgan Pure
  (Paterson)

Alumina
Baryta carb.
Calcarea carb.
Calcarea sulph.
Carbo veg.
Carboneum sulph.
Digitalis
Ferrum carb.
Medorrhinum
Psorinum
Tuberculinum bov.

Graphites
Kalium carb.
Magnesium carb.
Natrium carb.
Petroleum
Sepia
SULPHUR

THE BOWEL NOSODES

(B) *Morgan Gaertner* (Paterson)	Chelidonium Chenopodium Helleborus Hepar sulph. Lachesis	*LYCOPODIUM* Mercurius sulph. Sanguinaria Taraxacum
Proteus (Bach)	Acidum mur. Ammonium mur. Aurum mur. Apis Baryta mur. Borax Conium Cuprum met.	Calcarea mur. Ferrum mur. Ignatia Kalium mur. Magnesium mur. *NATRIUM MUR.* Secale
MUTABILE (Bach)	Ferrum phos. Kalium sulph. *PULSATILLA*	
BACILUS No. "7" (Paterson)	Arsenicum iod. Bromium Calcarea iod. Ferrum iod. *IODIUM* Kalium bich.	Kalium brom. *KALIUM CARB.* Kalium iod. Kalium nit. Mercurius iod. Natrium iod.
Gaertner (Bach)	Calcarea fluor. Calcarea hypophos. Calcarea phos. Calcarea sil. Kalium phos. Mercurius viv. Natrium phos. Syphilinum	Natrium sil. fluor. *PHOSPHORUS* Phytolacca Pulsatilla *SILICEA* Zincum phos.
DYS. Co. (Bach)	Anacardium Argentum nit. *ARSENICUM ALB.* Cadmium met.	Kalmia Veratrum album Veratrum viride

SYCOTIC Co. (Peterson)	Acidum nit. Antimonium tart. Calcarea metal. Ferrum met. Bacillinum	Natrium sulph. Rhus tox. *THUJA*
Faecalis (Bach)	*SEPIA*	

INDEX

A

Abrotanum 2, 10, 77, 158, 159, 163, 169, 219, 235, 273, 281, 313, 329, 338

Acetic acic 23, 35, 36, 46, 131, 169, 182, 261, 320

Aconitum napellus 2, 44, 48, 57, 59, 69, 78, 79, 101, 107, 109, 116, 147, 156, 157, 162, 175, 219, 220, 235, 239, 240, 256, 272, 275, 281, 303, 304, 305, 310, 338

Aesculus hippocastanum 9, 24, 111, 112, 182, 327

Aethusa cynapium 1, 6, 331

Agaricus muscarius 1, 7, 8, 17, 117, 123, 173, 180, 183, 218, 245, 264, 290, 301, 318, 331, 338, 429, 442, 443

Agnus castus 40, 137, 175

Ailanthus glandulosa 22, 110, 112, 127

Aletris farinosa 92, 149

Allium cepa 23, 47, 78, 87, 134, 160, 175, 237, 244

Aloe socotrina 9, 16, 32, 40, 49, 69, 75, 112, 119, 200, 215, 220, 240, 253, 254, 256, 262, 271, 280, 286, 307, 309, 325

Alumen 64, 142, 226, 321

Alumina 6, 7, 24, 38, 40, 50, 56, 57, 70, 74, 87, 89, 101, 107, 136, 150, 159, 163, 164, 196, 197, 201, 225, 238, 243, 250, 252, 258, 281, 287, 289, 313, 334, 338

Ammonium carbonicum 3, 44, 47, 64, 66, 91, 150, 166, 167, 173, 176, 186, 220, 231, 276, 293, 334, 341

Ammonium muriaticum 17, 39, 95, 190, 192, 221

Ambra grisea 12, 275, 325

INDEX

Amylenum nitrosum. 3, 40, 58, 73, 135, 141, 202, 251

Anacardium orientale 19, 50, 52, 81, 82, 107, 135, 148, 165, 175, 178, 181, 228, 237, 251, 256, 300, 329

Anisum stellatum 322

Antimonium crudum 11, 21, 24, 31, 32, 76, 88, 102, 143, 160, 162, 202, 217, 230, 293, 306, 326

Antimonium tartaricum 12, 30, 33, 67, 86, 90, 102, 107, 161, 162, 164, 180, 184, 186, 227, 256, 324

Anthracinum 29, 45, 91, 117, 319

Apis 8, 10, 34, 35, 36, 37, 39, 44, 58, 63, 66, 84, 86, 89, 110, 122, 127, 132, 146, 147, 170, 172, 177, 219, 221, 222, 228, 234, 236, 242, 243, 247, 269, 270, 276, 284, 286, 305, 319, 320, 329, 455, 471

Apocynum cannabinum 35, 37, 69, 147, 337

Aralia racemosa 164

Aranea diadema 32, 130, 222, 224

Argentum metallicum 286

Argentrum nitricum 18, 25, 27, 30, 48, 49, 52, 82, 89, 105, 107, 112, 120, 139, 150, 178, 182, 196, 248, 273, 274, 310, 321

Arnica montana 2, 3, 21, 44, 54, 55, 62, 79, 93, 94, 95, 106, 115, 133, 134, 144, 145, 146, 147, 154, 155, 167, 181, 196, 212, 213, 235, 256, 258, 262, 265, 270, 272, 273, 298, 311, 312, 321, 334

Arsenicum iodatum 14, 224

Arsenicum album 3, 10, 11, 14, 16, 26, 28, 29, 32, 35, 36, 37, 40, 41, 46, 47, 55, 62, 63, 64, 65, 71, 75, 78, 84, 87, 91, 97, 99, 100, 106, 110, 115, 120, 121, 122, 127, 130, 132, 138, 145, 147, 151, 162, 167, 171, 175, 184, 187, 191, 194, 197, 204, 210, 216, 219, 225, 226, 233, 242, 249, 252, 256, 257, 260, 263, 268, 280, 281, 284, 290, 296,

INDEX

299, 307, 309, 310, 311, 317, 319, 320, 321, 322, 326, 333, 334, 341, 352, 368, 393, 395, 417, 446, 448, 452

Arum dracontium 276

Arum triphyllum 38, 40, 129, 147, 175

Asafoetida 13, 20, 52, 53, 176, 177, 178, 209, 314, 331

Asarum europaeum 40, 64, 72, 73, 91, 135, 177, 197, 314, 330, 331, 341

Astacus fluviatilis 156

Asterrias rubens 114, 115

Aurum metallicum 39, 41, 69, 77, 114, 172, 175, 205, 216, 250, 267, 300, 301, 314

B

Badiaga 87, 99, 167

Baptisia tinctoria 42, 44, 56, 126, 127, 140, 228, 262, 272, 304

Baryta carbonica 19, 54, 57, 67, 134, 143, 146, 150, 192, 195, 233, 256, 268, 281, 291

Bellis perennis 133, 181, 279

Belladonna 3, 8, 11, 16, 21, 25, 35, 51, 53, 66, 70, 76, 82, 86, 90, 93, 97, 98, 108, 109, 128, 130, 131, 133, 140, 141, 146, 147, 154, 163, 172, 174, 189, 193, 194, 201, 202, 205, 232, 234, 236, 245, 253, 258, 271, 279, 290, 303, 304, 305, 310, 328, 331, 337, 341

Benzoicum acidum 253

Berberis vulgaris 60, 77, 132, 186, 198, 282, 283, 286, 293, 316, 321

Bismuth 50, 97, 109, 167, 185, 302, 304

Borax. 66, 67, 97, 98, 106, 115, 135, 139, 143, 171, 175, 186, 258, 279, 281, 282, 298, 310, 311, 329

Bovista 22, 23, 34, 44, 64, 72, 84, 115, 166, 171, 175, 192, 219, 272, 293, 304, 334, 429, 430

Bromium 12, 43, 68, 87, 143, 159, 160, 163, 164, 176, 260, 297

Bryonia 2, 16, 19, 27, 31, 36, 55, 58, 59, 62, 65, 72, 76, 86, 96,
   97, 98, 100, 102, 107, 109, 110, 111, 128, 130, 131, 133,
   134, 147, 167, 168, 174, 176, 178, 190, 193, 194, 216,
   222, 223, 229, 232, 233, 234, 235, 237, 240, 243, 246,
   250, 252, 260, 261, 265, 267, 268, 269, 270, 274, 304,
   308, 310, 318, 334, 335, 337, 429

Bufo rana 121, 173, 201

C

Cactus grandiflorus 25, 27, 66, 112, 123, 159, 169, 182, 183,
   193, 196, 202, 216, 295, 296

Caladium 13, 14, 40, 64, 86, 226, 257, 286, 287

Calcarea fluorica 78

Calcarea iodide 57

Calcarea phosphorica 30, 40, 61, 79, 80, 94, 104, 148, 156,
   219, 225, 239, 240, 293, 312, 327, 328

Calcarea carbonica 11, 12, 15, 18, 20, 29, 51, 53, 55, 56, 57, 65,
   66, 72, 76, 77, 78, 87, 92, 115, 116, 124, 129, 131, 143,
   144, 146, 151, 159, 164, 175, 176, 185, 187, 192, 193,
   197, 202, 213, 218, 219, 221, 227, 238, 239, 244, 253,
   254, 260, 261, 266, 267, 268, 275, 279, 280, 281, 286,
   288, 291, 292, 294, 298, 300, 309, 322, 329

Calendula 64, 91, 145, 146, 155, 292, 311, 312

Camphora 90, 150, 196, 200, 260, 284, 334, 341

Cannabis indica 12, 18, 39, 107, 121, 196, 228, 239, 321

Cannabis sativa 27, 321, 326

Cantharides 36, 61, 62, 83, 91, 109, 110, 132, 164, 189, 238,
   239, 247, 264, 275, 286, 321, 326, 341, 430

Capsicum 83, 104, 202

INDEX

Carbolic acid 27, 28, 29, 110, 127, 139, 164, 174, 225, 262, 263, 264, 295

Carbo animalis 19, 51, 67, 78, 84, 107, 142, 159, 166, 180, 200, 218, 237, 334

Carbo vegetabilis 46, 54, 81, 86, 87, 90, 91, 92, 94, 95, 103, 104, 116, 136, 168, 171, 173, 174, 186, 187, 196, 225, 233, 263, 333, 334

Carduus marianus 99, 104

Cascarilla 99, 176

Caulophyllum 7, 8, 95, 192, 193, 194, 275, 302, 429

Causticum 5, 19, 20, 24, 40, 48, 49, 50, 66, 67, 72, 88, 89, 97, 106, 108, 109, 114, 121, 123, 127, 137, 139, 144, 151, 167, 173, 175, 182, 198, 201, 212, 220, 221, 224, 233, 243, 271, 282, 298, 300, 303, 306, 313, 331, 442

Chamomilla 8, 42, 58, 98, 102, 108, 109, 112, 157, 169, 189, 192, 194, 230, 234, 249, 266, 267, 305, 331, 338

Chelidonium 27, 100, 124, 133, 167, 193, 204, 205, 235, 237, 251, 254, 269, 279, 289, 298, 318, 334

Chenopodium glaucum 98

China 37, 44, 82, 88, 90, 115, 123, 124, 136, 150, 158, 166, 186, 187, 197, 239, 241, 242, 244, 253, 260, 277, 328, 334

Chininum sulphuricum 103, 104, 163, 177, 199, 322, 338

Chlorine 67, 127, 277, 286

Cicuta virosa 18, 59, 102, 304

Cimicifuga (Act-sp.) 12, 20, 69, 75, 82, 92, 93, 114, 123, 145, 175, 183, 192, 264, 295, 429, 442

Cimex 24, 95

Cina 63, 86, 96, 102, 129, 153, 159, 176, 187, 256, 265, 273, 286, 295, 320

Cinnabaris 210

Cinnmomum 177

Clematis 196, 265, 267, 317

Cobaltum 337, 338, 429

Coccus cacti 128, 129, 159

Coca 20, 25, 105, 106, 124, 135, 137, 138

Cocaine 124

Coccculus 7, 19, 38, 87, 92, 94, 100, 109, 110, 120, 123, 135, 142, 159, 179, 189, 225, 226, 227, 228, 229, 230, 236, 237, 238, 334

Coffea cruda 42, 62, 94, 96, 97, 98, 138, 156, 157, 158, 177, 194, 223, 260, 324

Colchicum 45, 60, 84, 161, 179, 228, 230, 267, 274, 290, 299, 302, 316, 320, 333

Collinsonia 9, 69, 254

Colocynthis 68, 104, 112, 114, 125, 126, 133, 166, 188, 190, 193, 194, 266, 268, 274, 299, 300, 303

Commocladia dentata 295

Conium maculatum 19, 37, 50, 51, 52, 57, 64, 73, 86, 97, 104, 130, 145, 148, 159, 160, 166, 171, 176, 177, 179, 181, 188, 190, 192, 205, 229, 245, 267, 273, 277, 293, 301, 329, 338

Convalaria 125

Copaiva 60, 223, 326

Coralium rubrum 128, 129, 152

Croccus sativus 123, 138, 156, 176, 228, 249, 250, 275, 309, 325, 331

Crotalus horridus 119, 145, 170, 173, 216, 226, 262, 284, 311, 319

INDEX

Crotalus tiglium 16, 28, 40, 51, 55, 71, 127, 136, 145, 181, 246, 293
Cubeba 83
Culex 325
Cundurango 47, 150
Cuprum metallicum 41, 57, 129, 200, 292, 293, 305, 334, 337
Curare 245, 442

D

Daphne 196
Digitalis 6, 36, 37, 72, 104, 112, 118, 139, 147, 159, 187, 210, 296, 336
Dioscoria 22, 112, 240
Diphtherinum 54
Drosera 20, 38, 153, 243, 271
Dulcamara 57, 115, 224

E

Elaps corallinus 116, 119, 316, 429
Epigea 178
Equisetum 84, 282
Erechthites 213
Erigeron canadensis 161
Eugenia jambos 166
Eupatorim perfoliatum 94, 133, 161, 196, 262
Eupatorium purpureum 133
Euphorbia 29
Euphrasia 14, 15, 136, 162, 219, 229, 273

F

Ferrrum phosphoricum 132, 136, 194, 201
Ferrum metallicum 2, 25, 49, 60, 104, 122, 123, 131, 134, 141, 149, 158, 199, 229, 253, 275, 278, 314, 330
Fluoricum acidum 56, 57, 64, 78, 105, 288, 294, 312

G

Gambogia 17, 51, 119, 120, 253, 284
Gelsemia 18, 39, 50, 54, 55, 59, 72, 83, 91, 92, 94, 95, 108, 124, 127, 141, 146, 164, 165, 188, 192, 200, 202, 235, 240, 245, 248, 317, 336, 341
Gettysburg 294
Glonoinum 21, 25, 53, 58, 59, 71, 73, 188, 202, 217, 336
Gnaphalium 113
Graphites 24, 56, 67, 75, 95, 130, 137, 139, 149, 166, 175, 180, 220, 225, 226, 235, 237, 247, 256, 259, 264, 279, 281, 288, 292, 293, 294, 313, 429
Gratiola 51, 119
Grindelia 173, 176, 235
Guajacum 95, 212, 221
Gymnocladia 163

H

Hamamelis 44, 55, 66, 154, 170, 181, 212, 213, 327, 429
Hecla lava 138
Helleborus 36, 58, 69, 80, 188, 234, 253, 320, 329, 337, 338
Helonias dioica 77, 80, 92, 97, 183, 200, 214, 429
Hepar sulphur 6, 22, 40, 48, 56, 57, 64, 67, 68, 69, 70, 74, 79, 80, 109, 135, 142, 143, 144, 160, 164, 168, 174, 176, 190, 198, 203, 205, 211, 220, 221, 226, 227, 229, 237,

247, 258, 265, 266, 268, 271, 281, 292, 293, 294, 297, 298, 302, 306, 310, 312, 328, 442

Hydrastis canadensis 146, 156, 163, 189, 197, 295, 318

Hyoscyamus 12, 20, 59, 69, 77, 82, 128, 154, 156, 165, 189, 234, 236, 271, 303, 304, 305, 333

I

Ignatia 9, 20, 35, 42, 77, 85, 94, 101, 107, 109, 116, 117, 135, 138, 139, 146, 158, 161, 163, 167, 172, 174, 176, 191, 222, 227, 228, 230, 232, 236, 239, 249, 250, 259, 300, 303, 304, 317, 324, 330, 331, 334, 338

Indigo 12, 128

Iodine 1, 2, 27, 30, 57, 67, 68, 78, 107, 114, 151, 164, 167, 169, 193, 219, 220, 222, 276, 281, 292, 298, 313, 329

Ipecacuanha 31, 33, 44, 49, 104, 122, 129, 136, 140, 184, 187, 200, 212, 233, 254, 266, 277, 301, 316, 317, 327, 334

J

Jalapa 175, 185, 254

Jatropha curcas 51, 80

K

Kali bichromicum 35, 62, 65, 75, 76, 84, 127, 139, 152, 160, 175, 176, 177, 182, 186, 209, 219, 228, 231, 246, 255, 259, 261, 429

Kali bromatum 114, 120, 293

Kali iodatum 223, 247, 289, 299, 314

Kali muriaticum 80, 208, 237, 256, 260, 261

Kali nitricum 60, 190

Kali phosphoricum 12, 27, 78, 138, 165, 247, 248, 249, 250, 256, 276, 294

Kali permanganicum 236

Kali sulphuricum 34, 131, 163, 168, 259

Kalmia 72, 140, 178, 180, 267, 293, 295, 296

Kreosotum 23, 91, 96, 102, 142, 171, 173, 178, 182, 190, 211, 242, 260, 266, 289, 301, 327

L

Lactic acid 2, 178, 205, 258

Lac caninum 6, 13, 26, 35, 49, 64, 67, 81, 114, 126, 127, 133, 148, 163, 173, 174, 181, 182, 183, 189, 190, 193, 194, 205, 228, 245, 246, 251, 259, 274, 280, 314, 330, 331, 429, 442

Lac defloratum 13, 115, 164, 176, 243, 255

Lachesis 3, 12, 14, 19, 21, 25, 28, 29, 31, 35, 36, 40, 41, 46, 65, 71, 72, 110, 116, 119, 120, 131, 140, 141, 147, 150, 156, 161, 164, 168, 169, 170, 174, 175, 176, 177, 181, 182, 186, 187, 188, 194, 197, 200, 202, 204, 205, 208, 213, 216, 217, 219, 220, 228, 235, 236, 242, 246, 247, 274, 276, 279, 281, 283, 289, 290, 297, 298, 304, 305, 313, 316, 317, 319, 320, 321, 322, 324, 328

Lachnanthes 24, 242

Lappa major 148

Laurocerasus 233, 257

Ledum palustre 43, 84, 87, 145, 154, 155, 169, 191, 200, 204, 218, 267, 282, 288, 292, 295, 311, 331

Leptandra 262

Lilium tigrinum 8, 26, 39, 51, 62, 66, 93, 116, 149, 175, 184, 185, 190, 214, 218, 220, 254, 263, 280, 290, 442

Lithium carbonicum 52, 60, 73

Lobelia 11, 230

INDEX 483

Lycopodium 13, 19, 27, 31, 41, 52, 61, 62, 64, 65, 67, 72, 76,
    93, 99, 100, 113, 114, 123, 131, 133, 136, 144, 150, 161,
    166, 167, 168, 174, 175, 176, 181, 187, 193, 194, 197,
    198, 202, 213, 228, 242, 253, 254, 256, 259, 260, 261,
    267, 274, 282, 283, 288, 294, 302, 303, 308, 309, 313,
    317, 322, 325, 334

Lyssinum 59, 60, 64, 135, 148, 163, 187, 214, 243, 245, 304,
    305, 325, 429

M

M-arct. 294

Magnesia carbonica 6, 10, 21, 66, 151, 182, 198, 265, 266, 310

Magnesia muriatica 23, 64, 178, 202, 220, 280, 293

Magnesia phosphorica 58, 90, 112, 133, 163, 188, 190, 236,
    260, 341

Magnesia sulphurica 66, 201

Manganum aceticum 259

Mang. 331

Medorrhinum 12, 13, 61, 80, 98, 129, 190, 236, 281, 282, 307,
    313, 324, 326, 429, 442, 443

Melilotus alba 58, 59, 141, 255, 256, 429

Menyantes 71

Mephitis 276, 277

Mercuris cyanatus 126, 127

Mercurius 2, 3, 20, 31, 39, 48, 49, 64, 84, 91, 95, 98, 99, 100,
    107, 113, 131, 133, 149, 160, 161, 176, 180, 183, 189,
    191, 192, 197, 205, 211, 212, 216, 219, 224, 225, 227,
    239, 246, 247, 254, 259, 282, 283, 293, 299, 308, 312,
    313, 314, 317, 326

Mercurius biniodatus 206

Mercurius corrosivus 207
Mercurius dulcis 208
Mercurius solubilis 209
Mercurius sulphuricus 210
Mezereum 204, 205, 256, 265, 301, 325, 429
Millefolium 2, 71, 161, 233, 272, 275, 327, 328, 429
Muriatic acid 9, 16, 17, 55, 56, 59, 220, 226, 241, 311, 320
Murex 177, 182, 183, 215, 218, 220, 248, 280, 287, 289, 290, 429
Mygale 11, 12, 216
Myrtus communis 75, 322

N

Naja tripudians 51, 119, 174, 295, 296, 319
Natrium carbonicum 4, 133, 140, 142, 175, 220, 222, 227, 236, 260, 266, 273, 307, 443
Natrium muriaticum 1, 16, 27, 31, 35, 39, 41, 77, 95, 133, 134, 146, 150, 159, 164, 168, 169, 174, 175, 188, 192, 197, 201, 203, 204, 218, 224, 225, 226, 237, 240, 247, 251, 257, 258, 269, 272, 273, 280, 281, 283, 287, 295, 298, 300, 317, 325, 329, 331, 442
Natrium phosphoricum 183, 209
Natrium sulphuricum 34, 60, 109, 130, 151, 209, 218, 229, 259, 270, 271
Niccolum 223, 260
Nitricum acidum 20, 26, 27, 40, 41, 48, 55, 76, 143, 150, 157, 168, 173, 174, 175, 179, 189, 205, 215, 219, 220, 221, 230, 262, 264, 275, 289, 294, 303, 311, 321, 326
Nitri spiritus dulcis 241
Nux moschata 6, 33, 106, 116, 156, 176, 230, 231, 259, 287, 298, 319, 321, 325

INDEX 485

Nux vomica 9, 11, 12, 17, 22, 27, 43, 51, 63, 68, 69, 70, 72, 73, 76, 94, 97, 100, 101, 106, 107, 109, 112, 117, 120, 143, 149, 151, 153, 154, 157, 158, 167, 175, 178, 186, 191, 201, 207, 214, 218, 234, 236, 241, 245, 252, 254, 260, 268, 276, 277, 290, 301, 304, 317, 318, 331, 334, 338, 348, 443

O

Ocimum 198

Oleander 16, 151, 220, 262, 271

Opium 2, 12, 19, 33, 44, 58, 59, 69, 81, 91, 97, 99, 108, 154, 173, 190, 227, 229, 251, 252, 262, 263, 281, 302, 304, 305, 334

Origanum 72, 214, 248

Oxalic acid 57, 77, 80, 148, 197, 200

P

Palladium 37

Paris quadrifolia 151, 202

Petroselinum 18, 55, 84, 164, 220, 248, 252, 293, 304

Petroleum 83, 95, 170

Phosphoric acid 13, 77, 94, 103, 138, 149, 166, 172, 241, 242, 243, 248, 250, 276, 287, 288, 300, 333

Phellandrinum 246

Phosphorus 12, 15, 20, 23, 24, 35, 38, 46, 48, 53, 65, 68, 70, 71, 76, 87, 88, 90, 94, 95, 102, 104, 116, 118, 120, 126, 136, 153, 154, 159, 166, 168, 169, 170, 171, 173, 177, 179, 185, 186, 190, 217, 233, 236, 241, 244, 247, 248, 250, 253, 255, 257, 264, 266, 271, 279, 280, 283, 284, 287, 289, 294, 298, 299, 300, 307, 317, 323, 330, 429, 443

Physostigma 155

Picric acid 84, 200, 209, 241, 250, 294

Pip-m. 27

Pix liquida 322

Plantago major 296, 317

Platina 18, 53, 69, 91, 169, 177, 183, 214, 228, 236, 252, 299, 302, 319, 325, 341, 442

Plumbum 90, 99, 104, 150, 194, 220, 235, 262, 334

Podophyllum 17, 49, 52, 54, 58, 60, 98, 99, 119, 124, 126, 133, 146, 151, 157, 193, 204, 220, 252, 266, 269, 271, 274, 299

Psorinum 12, 15, 16, 18, 19, 24, 27, 54, 56, 57, 64, 65, 77, 78, 79, 80, 87, 88, 91, 95, 101, 115, 143, 149, 150, 151, 160, 166, 175, 178, 185, 187, 197, 203, 221, 222, 236, 262, 263, 265, 266, 273, 278, 279, 281, 282, 286, 291, 292, 293, 306, 307, 308, 309, 311, 314, 316, 329, 330, 341, 351, 429, 442, 443

Ptelea trifoliata 68, 70

Pulsatilla 6, 7, 8, 10, 14, 15, 19, 23, 24, 27, 30, 31, 33, 34, 35, 39, 40, 49, 50, 62, 68, 69, 70, 73, 75, 76, 86, 90, 92, 93, 94, 98, 104, 109, 117, 122, 123, 129, 132, 134, 142, 144, 145, 158, 160, 162, 163, 175, 177, 178, 180, 192, 193, 194, 202, 204, 219, 220, 222, 223, 227, 228, 229, 231, 233, 239, 241, 244, 245, 246, 249, 250, 254, 271, 274, 276, 280, 287, 288, 290, 293, 298, 303, 309, 310, 311, 321, 322, 324, 330, 337, 429, 442

Pyrogenum 28, 29, 42, 44, 46, 54, 55, 91, 118, 119, 133, 174, 228, 235, 272, 305, 320, 430, 442

R

Ranunculus bulbosus 7, 11, 31, 70, 87, 274, 303

Ranunculus scleratus 143, 318

INDEX

Ratanhia 157, 225, 226

Rheum 1, 7, 61, 74, 77, 92, 95, 151, 163, 169, 179, 190, 199, 229, 267, 278, 282, 295, 310, 311, 314, 345, 404, 406, 427, 428, 429, 432, 439

Rhododendron 37, 169, 229, 268, 270, 443

Rhus radicans 27

Rhus toxicodendron 15, 27, 31, 35, 36, 39, 42, 44, 52, 57, 62, 66, 67, 70, 93, 94, 97, 99, 115, 119, 120, 126, 131, 150, 163, 177, 180, 190, 202, 204, 206, 212, 216, 229, 240, 244, 245, 246, 259, 263, 265, 267, 270, 272, 277, 304, 309, 310, 314, 318, 325, 337

Rhus venenata 27, 278

Robinia 310

Rumex 16, 95, 128

Ruta graveolens 39, 44, 78, 155, 157, 181, 272, 294, 311, 318

S

Sabadilla 274, 278

Sabina 4, 6, 7, 116, 142, 212, 217, 274, 276, 284, 288, 303, 326, 327

Salicylic acid 79, 265, 335

Sambucus nigra 22, 47, 129, 186, 199, 231, 326

Sanguinaria 15, 98, 100, 139, 141, 172, 176, 178, 193, 199, 202, 237, 271, 281, 282, 290, 295, 307, 314, 336, 429

Sanginaria nitrate 15, 278

Sanicula 1, 2, 11, 24, 32, 56, 63, 64, 65, 74, 75, 78, 97, 135, 139, 159, 192, 219, 221, 236, 237, 238, 251, 262, 266, 281, 286, 290, 292, 294, 306, 307, 325

Santoninum 102

Sarsaparilla 293

INDEX

Secale cornutum 29, 39, 47, 80, 81, 92, 93, 116, 150, 173, 180, 196, 200, 263, 275, 276, 305, 329, 429, 430

Selenium 13, 14, 40, 48, 72, 75, 104, 280, 324

Senecio aureus 272

Sepia 8, 13, 19, 20, 45, 53, 59, 66, 69, 75, 87, 92, 93, 95, 99, 100, 109, 110, 131, 133, 139, 142, 143, 146, 151, 156, 163, 170, 172, 175, 177, 178, 180, 182, 183, 202, 213, 214, 218, 220, 233, 250, 261, 264, 267, 283, 286, 292, 294, 298, 299, 309, 317, 328, 331, 333, 429, 442, 443

Silicea 15, 18, 19, 22, 24, 30, 40, 51, 54, 56, 57, 61, 64, 65, 74, 75, 76, 77, 78, 96, 102, 120, 121, 126, 138, 139, 146, 150, 151, 165, 178, 180, 192, 193, 203, 219, 222, 235, 237, 240, 241, 242, 246, 247, 248, 260, 261, 266, 271, 273, 278, 279, 280, 281, 282, 286, 291, 295, 300, 312, 321, 324, 325, 326, 331, 442, 443

Sinapis 323

Spigelia 47, 102, 169, 183, 216, 220, 273, 278, 293, 304, 310, 313, 320, 331

Spongia 3, 5, 67, 68, 102, 121, 136, 138, 160, 216, 271, 296, 298, 300, 302, 305

Scilla 31

Squilla 94, 220

Stannum 38, 93, 121, 124, 168, 236, 241, 243, 249, 250, 286, 287, 295, 309, 312

Staphysagria 44, 52, 63, 69, 102, 109, 112, 113, 125, 138, 155, 157, 161, 185, 220, 226, 240, 243, 249, 260, 265, 266, 287, 303, 314, 316, 325, 326

Sticta 22, 163, 330

Stramonium 12, 26, 58, 59, 63, 65, 82, 141, 154, 166, 173, 180, 188, 189, 236, 305, 333

Strontium 176, 192, 272

Sulphuric acid 2, 12, 44, 49, 50, 73, 79, 136, 252, 260, 314, 320

Sulphur 9, 12, 16, 18, 19, 21, 24, 25, 27, 30, 31, 40, 43, 46, 49, 51, 57, 62, 65, 67, 70, 74, 75, 76, 78, 87, 89, 90, 91, 95, 98, 100, 109, 112, 116, 117, 126, 129, 139, 143, 144, 147, 157, 159, 170, 171, 172, 173, 174, 177, 178, 181, 185, 187, 189, 190, 193, 197, 200, 204, 205, 210, 213, 224, 225, 231, 232, 233, 237, 241, 242, 254, 256, 258, 260, 261, 264, 265, 266, 270, 271, 277, 278, 279, 280, 281, 288, 289, 290, 291, 295, 300, 309, 311, 314, 322, 325, 328, 329, 330, 331, 333, 334, 337, 341, 429, 442, 443

Symphytum 42, 77, 79, 138, 272, 273, 311

Syphilinum 6, 19, 201, 325, 443

T

Tabacum 32, 34, 61, 62, 72, 158, 177, 183, 184, 200, 295, 301, 321, 332, 333, 334, 336

Taraxacum 204, 219

Tarentula 12, 33, 49, 53, 72, 117, 135, 174, 183, 333, 338, 442

Tellurium 280, 289

Terebinthina 32, 33, 55, 262, 311

Teucrium 15, 102, 163, 186, 209, 278, 294

Theridion 12, 53, 77, 191, 319, 324, 330, 338

Thlaspi 92, 93, 327, 328

Thuja 15, 20, 35, 46, 60, 116, 119, 121, 131, 132, 157, 181, 209, 220, 224, 226, 227, 235, 264, 274, 275, 280, 282, 292, 301, 303, 309, 314, 321, 322, 429, 442, 443

Trillium pendulum 275

INDEX

Tuberculinum 1, 2, 22, 46, 57, 64, 74, 75, 78, 137, 146, 147, 150, 159, 173, 254, 256, 257, 258, 276, 290, 300, 307, 308, 314, 330, 337, 338, 351, 442

U

Urtica urens 221, 429

Ustilago 7, 116, 117, 240, 290, 323, 325, 327, 328

V

Valeriana 20, 89, 90, 123, 233, 237, 250

Variolinum 331

Veratrum viride 279

Veratrum 19, 22, 33, 41, 44, 46, 63, 80, 81, 90, 94, 119, 122, 129, 143, 154, 157, 181, 184, 196, 200, 202, 203, 232, 260, 263, 288, 315, 316, 331

Verbascum 128

Viburnum opulus 429

X

Xanthoxylum 107

Z

Zincum 12, 14, 22, 34, 72, 117, 121, 122, 142, 147, 165, 173, 177, 194, 199, 200, 214, 233, 235, 236, 242, 248, 250, 252, 307, 318, 443

Zingiber 260